BIBLE HEALTH SECRETS

By Best-Selling Author of THE BIBLE CURE

REGINALD CHERRY, M.D.

SILOAM®

BIBLE HEALTH SECRETS by Reginald Cherry, M.D.
Published by Siloam
A part of Strang Communications Company
600 Rinehart Road
Lake Mary, Florida 32746
www.siloam.com

Unless otherwise noted, all Scripture quotations are from the King James Version of the Bible.

Scripture quotations marked AMP are from the Amplified Bible. Old Testament copyright © 1965, 1987 by the Zondervan Corporation. The Amplified New Testament copyright © 1954, 1958, 1987 by the Lockman Foundation. Used by permission.

Scripture quotations marked NIV are from the Holy Bible, New International Version. Copyright © 1973, 1978, 1984, International Bible Society. Used by permission.

Scripture quotations marked NKJV are from the New King James Version of the Bible. Copyright © 1979, 1980, 1982 by Thomas Nelson, Inc., publishers. Used by permission.

Scripture quotations marked NLT are from the Holy Bible, New Living Translation, copyright © 1996. Used by permission of Tyndale House Publishers, Inc., Wheaton, IL 60189. All rights reserved.

Scripture quotations marked TLB are from The Living Bible. Copyright © 1971. Used by permission of Tyndale House Publishers, Inc., Wheaton, IL 60189. All rights reserved.

Cover design by Larry Smith & Associates, Inc., Atlanta, GA

Library of Congress Cataloging-in-Publication Data

Cherry, Reginald B.
  Bible health secrets / Reginald Cherry.
      p. cm.
  Includes bibliographical references.
  ISBN 0-88419-937-1
  1. Medicine, Popular. 2. Health--Religious aspects--Christianity.
  3. Naturopathy. 4. Alternative medicine. I. Title.
RC82.C453 2003
615.5--dc21
                            2003007712

03 04 05 06 07 — 87654321
Printed in the United States of America

TABLE OF
CONTENTS

SPIRITUAL SECRETS FOR HEALTH AND HEALING

CHAPTER 1

YOUR UNIQUE
PATHWAY TO HEALING

*Don't be impressed with your own wisdom. Instead,
fear the LORD and turn your back on evil. Then you
will gain renewed health and vitality.*
—PROVERBS 3:7–8, NLT

S O MANY PEOPLE IN THE WORLD TODAY ARE SICK. Virtually none of us will remain untouched by illness, whether it affects our own bodies or the health of those we love. When we are healthy, we give little thought to the way our bodies function, even though that is the time we should be taking steps to maintain our health. Often we wait until we are sick or until some health crisis occurs to make the lifestyle changes necessary to reclaim our health.

You may have picked up this book for a number of reasons. More than likely, you or someone you love is suffering from some illness or disease, and you may be asking yourself, *Does God really want to see me healed?* Or you may already believe that God will heal you, but you may be wondering why He hasn't healed you in a particular way.

Let me answer the question once and for all: *God wants to heal you!* God desires for His people to be healthy and whole, certainly for their own benefit, but also to be able to take His light to a lost and dying world. However, many people seek for their healing to take place in a certain

1

way; most of them prefer it to happen instantaneously, without any real effort on their own part.

Perhaps instead of asking, "Why hasn't God healed me this way?", a better question would be, "Is there something that I'm doing to prevent my healing from taking place? Should I be doing something more than what I am doing now to facilitate my getting well?"

God has a unique pathway for every person, including a pathway to healing. And while I believe in instantaneous healing and wholeheartedly rejoice when such healing takes place, most of the time, God's pathway to healing takes place over a period of time as you walk in obedience to what He tells you to do. Sometimes that involves medical science; other times it incorporates the amazing natural substances that God has placed in His earth for the benefit and healing of His people. New scientific discoveries are taking place all the time that demonstrate that the very substances we need to walk in health exist within nature.

How I Became a Christian Doctor

I am a medical doctor who believes in the healing power of God, but that was not always the case. As a young man, I was drawn to watch Billy Graham's crusades on television, but that was about the extent of my spirituality. I had always had the desire to help people, and I knew from a very young age that I wanted to be a doctor and do what I could to eliminate sickness and disease from the world.

I attended medical school at one of the most godless institutions I had ever encountered—not because the people there were evil, but because they glorified science, reason and knowledge above all else. Physicians were trained to focus only on the body and perhaps the mind of the patient, but never the spirit—that was left up to the patient's minister or the chaplain on call.

Even so, I was fascinated in medical school with the sheer magnificence of the human body. Now I can express that fascination in the words of Scripture, which declares that we are "fearfully and wonderfully made" (Ps. 139:14). The body has such intricate systems, all working together as a whole; I realized that our bodies are too amazing to have simply evolved on their own from a one-cell organism millions of years ago. There had to be the hand of a Creator involved.

After completing medical school and my internship, I began seeing patients and discovered that they had real problems, many of which had stumped the medical community. There was only so much that doctors knew to do for many of the critical diseases that people faced.

I finally accepted Jesus Christ in 1979 and was born again. Through this life-changing experience, I discovered a whole new perspective on this business of making people whole. I began to see that there had to be a source of healing that surpassed what science and medicine had to offer. *Jehovah-Rapha* began to reveal to me that He is the source of all healing, whether it comes by natural or supernatural means. Around this time, I was privileged to observe several healings take place that resulted from the direct touch of God. Although I was skeptical at first, when I observed that the symptoms did not return to these persons' lives, I began to understand the power that God has to heal. I realized that He greatly desires to bless His children with healthy bodies and longevity in life.

I grew to accept the truth that God heals today, both naturally and miraculously. And then I began to apply that truth in my medical practice. As I began to seek with my patients the pathway to healing God had designed just for them, I watched people's lives change before my eyes. More and more patients began to walk in health, released from their diseases and free to do what God had called them to do.

God does not want any one of us to suffer needlessly under the curse of disease! It was never His intention for mankind to live under the oppression of sin and the consequences—such as illness—that sin brought into the world. But even after man's fall, God, in His great compassion, made provision for the health of His people. His care for the people of Israel in the Old Testament foreshadows the healing provision He has made for us today.

Health Secrets of the Old Covenant

In the Book of Exodus, the Lord recorded a wonderful promise for the health of His people. He declared that He would place "none of these diseases" on His people (Exod. 15:26). We understand that to mean that none of the diseases that plagued the people of that time would enter the camp of the Israelites—that is, as long as they kept the commandments of the Lord. These commandments are timeless; they still hold true for us today. Perhaps one of the greatest secrets the Bible holds for modern man is that the dietary laws of the Old Testament hold great significance for our health and well-being today.

Jesus' death on the cross purchased our healing once and for all, but that does not mean that the dietary laws God had already provided no longer have any meaning. In fact, these ancient Hebrew documents hold fascinating truths about medicine, health and hygiene that were centuries before their time. Modern medicine continues to prove that the teachings and the health codes given to the Israelites have great value for our health.

God introduced Himself to His people in the Old Testament as *Jehovah-Rapha*, the God who heals. Centuries before Christ died on the cross to purchase our salvation and healing, God was interested in the health of His people! Listen to His promise:

> *Worship the LORD your God, and his blessing will be on your food and water. I will take away sickness from among you, and none will miscarry or be barren in your land. I will give you a full life span.*
>
> —EXODUS 23:25–26, NIV

God's promise for His people still holds true for us today. But notice in this passage that He ties the blessings of good health, fertility and longevity of life to the blessing that is placed on what they put into their mouths—their food and water. Some people believe that this verse means they can simply speak a blessing, or "say grace," over a meal full of fat, sugar and carbohydrates, and their health will somehow be protected because the food has been "blessed." But what this promise is actually telling us is that God has directly tied what we eat and drink to the maintenance of health in our bodies.

I am convinced that before we receive our healing, we must obey God's commands as to what we should eat and drink. When we choose to follow what He tells us to do, we can begin to walk in the health and blessings He has planned for us. Throughout this book, we will explore some of the health secrets that can be found in the dietary laws of the Old Testament and learn how they relate to the most common and destructive ailments that we face in our lives today. Some of these health secrets include:

- Prohibitions against fatty foods

- Prohibitions against eating blood, which has the tendency to carry infection

- Healthy foods that increase longevity and help prevent disease

- Foods to avoid in order to maintain a healthy lifestyle

Proverbs 3:7–8 tells us, "Don't be impressed with your own wisdom. Instead, fear the LORD and turn your back on evil. Then you will regain renewed health and vitality" (NLT). In today's culture, eating the wrong foods isn't something that we would necessarily call evil. However, it can bring evil things, such as disease, into our lives. If we are willing to change our diets and follow God's commands, our health can be renewed! I encourage you to keep an open mind as we explore the dietary and health laws God gave to protect His people from disease.

Health Secrets of the New Covenant

In the New Testament, God continues to provide healing for His people. Jesus Christ came to earth and, through His sacrificial death on the cross, provided redemption for man, including eternal salvation from sin as well as healing from disease. The prophet Isaiah had foretold this wonderful redemption hundreds of years earlier:

> *But he was wounded for our transgressions, he was bruised for our iniquities: the chastisement of our peace was upon him; and with his stripes we are healed.*
> —ISAIAH 53:5

Throughout His life on earth, Jesus healed all manner of disease. There are many verses that tell us the magnitude of His healing ministry, such as this one:

> *But when Jesus knew it, he withdrew himself from thence: and great multitudes followed him, and he healed them all.*
> —MATTHEW 12:15

It is important to notice that, though Jesus healed multitudes of people, He did so in a variety of ways. There are times when a touch or a word from Jesus healed an infirm person instantly. (See Luke 4:39–40; 6:10.) But not as commonly understood by many people is the fact that sometimes Jesus used *natural substances* through which He caused His healing power to flow.

The most striking example of this method can be found in the Gospel of John, which relates the dramatic healing of a blind man:

> *As he went along, he saw a man blind from birth...He spit on the ground, made some mud with the saliva, and put it on the man's eyes. "Go," he told him, "wash in the Pool of Siloam."...So the man went and washed, and came home seeing.*
> —JOHN 9:1, 6–7, NIV

As this passage indicates, healing can take place instantaneously or as a process that occurs over a period of time. In this case, Jesus touched the blind man's eyes as He placed the mud solution on him, but the man was not healed at that time. His healing was complete when he followed Jesus' instructions and washed his eyes in the Pool of Siloam.

So many dear Christians today become disheartened if, after much prayer and petition to the throne of God, they do not receive instant, miraculous healing from their illness. But look carefully at what caused this man's healing recorded in John 9. First, he received a touch from Jesus. Then he accepted the application of a natural substance onto the diseased part of his body. And finally, he obeyed Jesus' unique instructions to him as an individual.

This blind man's experience explains for us one of the greatest health secrets of the Bible, one that is often overlooked by well-meaning Christians. I believe it is a vitally important truth that we need to understand in order to walk in the divine health that God would have for us. That truth is the wonderful secret that *God has a unique pathway to healing just for you.*

Let me state it another way: God heals different people in different ways. Some may attend a healing crusade and receive an instant miracle from the Lord. But more commonly, God will work through the natural substances that He has provided for us—namely, various foods, vitamins, minerals and even medications—to work out His healing plan. Sometimes He uses a combination of natural and supernatural methods to effect a cure. The key lies in discovering God's plan for *your own life.* It is not enough to expect what you may have seen occur in the lives of other Christians.

The story of the blind man is in the Bible for a very important reason. There are many other stories of miraculous, instantaneous healings that Jesus performed. But in this story, God is challenging us to seek Him for our own pathway to healing. Consider the following important conclusions we can safely draw from the account of the blind man's healing:

- The blind man wasn't healed when Jesus first touched him.

- Even so, at the moment of the touch, the healing process had begun.

- The blind man couldn't necessarily sense the healing process at that time.

- For the process to continue, the man had to listen to and carefully follow Jesus' instructions to him as an individual.

~ Jesus specifically told him the path to walk on (literally), the name of the pool to which he was to go and what he was to do when he got there.

~ As the man was obedient to Jesus' commands, his eyesight was fully restored.

Finding the Path God Has for You

Wherever I share the gospel and in whatever materials I write, I will always make the hearer and reader aware of what God taught me about the particular pathway to healing He has for each person. God's pathway to healing is available to each of us as we follow His ways and listen to His voice. As you seek for healing, I encourage you to begin to pray this prayer:

> *Father,*
> *I come to You, knowing that You desire to make my body whole. Please show me the path I must take to see the full manifestation of healing in my body.*

Once you have prayed, begin to allow Jehovah-Rapha to speak to you and make your pathway to healing clear. Be still before Him, and listen. God's Word promises that we can hear His voice, a reality to which many Bible heroes attest. Understand that from the minute you pray this prayer, the process has begun whether or not you see any immediate change.

Daniel experienced this phenomenon in the Old Testament when he prayed for twenty-one days, crying out to God for an answer on behalf of the people. When the angel of the Lord finally arrived, he told Daniel that from the moment he had begun to pray, the heavenly forces had been set in motion, even though Daniel couldn't see anything taking place in the natural realm. In the supernatural realm, however, the angel had to battle through the opposition to reach Daniel. (See Daniel 10.) So don't give up! Keep praying for your answer. Continue to seek God for His direction, and then when He gives it, be obedient to His commands.

Many times, God directs His people to the natural substances that He has already placed within His plant kingdom. Most of the directions that are given throughout this book refer to these amazing natural substances that God gave to man:

> *Then God said, "I give you every seed-bearing plant on the face*

*of the whole earth and every tree that has fruit with seed in it.
They will be yours for food."*

—GENESIS 1:29, NIV

We are a generation that is different from any other that has walked the face of the earth. Instead of eating food as it naturally comes from the earth, we eat food that our culture has determined has been affected by herbicides and pesticides of every kind. The air that we breathe is full of pollutants. The ozone layer is being depleted day by day. We are witnessing the fulfillment of Bible prophecy:

> *[In the last days] there will be mighty and violent earthquakes, and in various places famines and pestilences (plagues: malignant and contagious or infectious epidemic diseases which are deadly and devastating); and there will be sights of terror and great signs from heaven.*
>
> —LUKE 21:11, AMP

But even though these malignant and contagious diseases are virtually surrounding us, God has given our generation the knowledge necessary to extract and concentrate the beneficial elements from the plant kingdom. Generations before us did not need this divine wisdom as desperately as ours does. As we receive this divine wisdom given to man by God, perhaps our children and future generations will not suffer the ravages of disease we are experiencing.

Divine Purpose for Good Health

Jesus has instructed us to be "the light of the world" (Matt. 5:14). He told us to "go and make disciples of all the nations, baptizing them in the name of the Father and the Son and the Holy Spirit" (Matt. 28:19, NIV). But when Christians are sick, fatigued or just dragging around, they don't have the strength or energy it takes to be the light of the world to people who need to know our Savior. They are not interested in going anywhere to share the good news of the gospel with those who desperately need to hear.

One of the most effective strategies of the enemy is to attack Christians in their bodies so that they can no longer carry out the work God has for them. Satan would love to see every one of God's people lying sick in their beds, focused only on themselves and their own pain and misery. Let's not allow him to succeed!

Don't just pursue your health so that you can be free of painful symptoms—seek God's pathway to healing so that you will be able to carry out His destiny for your life with strength, vigor and power! Don't allow the devil to cut your life short with a terminal illness or steal another precious day from your divine destiny simply because you are sick or fatigued.

As you read this book, continue to pray that God will show you what things He would have you to do to improve your health, perhaps even using the healing elements that already exist in His natural kingdom. I encourage you to find your own pathway to healing so that you can carry His light to a lost and dying world. Decide which of the health secrets we are going to discuss may apply to your situation.

ASK DR. CHERRY

QUESTION: **I have just received a negative report from the doctor. What should I do?**

ANSWER: When a person receives a negative report or a poor diagnosis from a physician, their first response is usually to panic, which can lead to feelings of despair. There are several truths from God's Word concerning disease on which you can focus to overcome these negative feelings:

1. *God loves you, and He wants you healed.* Meditate on such passages as Exodus 15:26; Isaiah 53; and 1 Peter 2:24. Read through the Gospels, and note especially the healings of Jesus. Our merciful God has provided the way for your healing through the shed blood of His Son; He does not want to see any of His children suffer needlessly under the curse of disease.

2. *You have been uniquely made.* Read and meditate on Psalm 139. God Himself carefully and lovingly formed your body within your mother's womb. If He took such time and care to form you, how much more will He continue to care for your body and provide the way for your healing to be completed?

3. *You have been uniquely attacked with disease.* Each person's illness is unique to them. Different genetic dispositions and factors combine in an individual's body to cause various diseases to occur.

4. *You have been given a unique pathway to healing.* Because you are an individual, and because God chooses to deal with each of us in His own way, there is a unique pathway to healing for you. God, in His perfect plan and His great love for you, has already made provision for the cure for your disease.

5. *Pray for the understanding of that pathway.* Through the guidance of the Holy Spirit, you can begin to understand what the pathway is that God has for your individual healing. This book may be part of your answer to help you discover other biblical secrets regarding your particular disease, which may guide you toward your own pathway to healing.

QUESTION: **There are so many diseases in the world, and some life-threatening diseases even run in my family. How should I deal with the fear that I might die of heart disease or cancer?**

ANSWER: Facing disease can be scary! But as Christians, we can confront our fears by standing on the promises of God. He tells us to "be strong and take heart, all you who hope in the Lord" (Ps. 31:24, NIV). Jesus comforts us with the following words: "Peace I leave with you, My peace I give to you; not as the world gives do I give to you. Let not your heart be troubled, neither let it be afraid" (John 14:27, NKJV). God's peace is available to His children, especially when they place their absolute trust in His care.

God made your body, and He knows how to fix it when things go wrong. Because He understands how the human body functions best, it is in our best interest to follow what He tells us to do. Eating right and taking the right nutrients that He has provided for us in the plant kingdom is one important step that you can take. You can confront your fears by firmly standing your ground in the Word of God, but also with the knowledge that you have taken the preventive measures necessary to protect your health—especially the recommendations given throughout this book. Do the things that you know to do, and then rest in His peace.

QUESTION: **Why is it that many people who are "instantly" healed in a healing crusade or service sometimes lose that healing?**

ANSWER: People who genuinely experience divine healing can lose their healing within a few weeks simply because they do not make the necessary lifestyle changes to maintain that healing. Let me use a medical healing process to give you an example of this sad reality. A person who has advanced heart disease because of poor eating habits and high cholesterol levels may have surgery to receive new bypass grafts. However, if there is no change in lifestyle, that person may face the exact same situation of advanced heart disease in a few months or years. In this same way, God in His mercy may heal someone, but only that person can make the decision to walk in divine health, following God's health laws and taking care of his or her body, thus maintaining the healing God gave.

CHAPTER 2

DIETARY LAWS
FOR TODAY

*Do not think that I have come to abolish the
Law or the Prophets; I have not come to
abolish them but to fulfill them.*
—MATTHEW 5:17, NIV

BUT I'M NOT UNDER THE LAW! I LIVE IN GRACE!" The burning questions most often asked whenever I share the benefits of following the Old Testament laws for health and hygiene go something like this:

- ∾ "But I'm not under the law! Why should I be concerned with dietary regulations that were established under the Mosaic Law for people living before Christ?"

- ∾ "The Old Testament is outdated and so hard to read. What relevance could it possibly have for my life today?"

- ∾ "Why should I follow the teachings of the Old Testament—especially the ones regarding health and diet? Hasn't Jesus already fulfilled the Law?"

As Christians, we have been taught in church that Christ fulfilled the Law, and that is true. Jesus Himself declared, "Do not think that I have come to abolish the Law or the Prophets; I have not come to abolish them but to fulfill them" (Matt. 5:17, NIV). But what does that mean? By virtue of His fulfilling the Law, did He mean they were no longer in effect—that they were abolished? He could not mean that, for that would contradict Jesus' own words. He did not come to abolish the Law or the prophets.

Are the Old Testament laws (recorded in Leviticus and Deuteronomy) no longer valid or useful? That cannot be the case, because Jesus said He hadn't abolished, or destroyed, the Law. There must still be something useful about it, some benefits we will reap for our lives today by keeping the laws of God. Then the question arises: If we decide to keep the Old Testament laws, shouldn't we also keep the sacrificial system, offering burnt offerings to God or having a priest make atonement for our sins? Confusion surrounding God's laws arises because of a lack of understanding them. We need to understand how Jesus fulfilled the Law through His life and through His death.

Because obedience to the Word of God is key to our healing and our health, we need to learn to hear His voice and understand His commands. That begins with searching the words He has already spoken in the Bible, God's written Word.

Under the Old Covenant

God gave the Law to His people, the Israelites, first on Mount Sinai with the giving of the Ten Commandments. Later as the Israelites wandered in the wilderness, God set forth, in miniscule detail, all of the specific laws that would govern every area of the people's lives.

Today we have trouble relating to all of the instructions given to the Israelites to establish their cultural life as a nation. For example, we wonder why God would require His people to purposely and unconditionally burn down any house that showed signs of mildew. Why did He allow people to eat beef but forbid their eating of pork? How could these regulations possibly apply to our lives today?

The fact is that the health and nutritional laws God gave to the Israelites thousands of years ago are some of the most advanced guidelines for avoiding plagues and disease that have ever been developed. Scientific studies are proving that the foods the Israelites were instructed to eat in the Old Testament contain curative properties, or substances that can prevent or even reverse disease. And the "unclean" animals they were forbidden to eat are those that carry the most dangerous bacteria and risk of disease even today. Another example of prohibition to the Israelites was the eating of blood. Now it is common knowledge in the medical community that the blood of animals can carry dangerous infections.

All of this proves that God doesn't just arbitrarily give laws to His people simply to amuse Himself or to prevent us from having a good time—they are always for our own good! It is important to understand that in the Mosaic Law there are three primary categories of regulations:

- The Ten Commandments, *moral laws,* which govern behavior and relationship with God and one another

- The sacrificial system, *ceremonial laws,* which govern daily operations of the temple and outline the function of the priests

- The social hygiene system, *health and dietary laws,* which help God's people prevent disease

Christians today are probably most familiar with the Ten Commandments, the moral laws, that were given on the stone tablets to Moses on Mount Sinai. These moral laws, such as "Thou shalt not kill," are still very much in effect for our lives today. In fact, Jesus took these laws to a new level when He declared that even carrying anger against your brother would put you in danger of judgment the same as murdering him would (Matt. 5:21–22). And with regards to the commandment "Thou shalt not commit adultery," Jesus declared that lusting after a woman was the same as committing adultery with her in your heart (Matt. 5:28). We cannot say that because Jesus fulfilled the Law we are free from these moral laws given under the Mosaic covenant.

There is nothing in Scripture that validates the notion that God's health and dietary laws were nullified either. In fact, as I have mentioned, we are beginning to understand the medical significance of these laws as they relate to our own health risks today. Like the moral laws, these dietary laws were given for our protection—not for our punishment, as many assume.

Regarding the ceremonial laws that established a priesthood and a system of sacrifice to atone for the sins of the people, they foreshadowed the coming work of Christ on the cross. Of course, because Christ completed—fulfilled—the redemptive work at Calvary, the Scriptures teach us clearly that we have a better sacrifice than that of bulls and goats. We receive by faith the sacrifice of Christ for the forgiveness of our sins. To continue the Mosaic sacrificial system would be to deny salvation through faith in Christ. The writer to the Hebrews states clearly:

But Christ being come an high priest of good things to come, by a greater and more perfect tabernacle, not made with hands, that is to say, not of this building; neither by the blood of goats and calves, but by his own blood he entered in once into the holy place, having obtained eternal redemption for us. For if the blood of bulls and of goats, and the ashes of an heifer sprinkling the unclean, sanctifieth to the purifying of the flesh: How much more shall the blood of Christ, who through the eternal Spirit offered himself without spot to God, purge your conscience from dead works to serve the living God?

—Hebrews 9:11–14

Having stated that the moral laws and the dietary laws that God gave His people are still in effect, we need to note an important difference between living under the Old Covenant and life for Christians under the New Covenant. For Israel, the keeping of every single law, in all three categories—even to the most minute of details—was required for righteousness. Keeping the Law determined a person's right standing with God.

Even if an Israelite kept all of the Ten Commandments but slipped up on a minor detail of the dietary laws, he was considered "unclean" in his relationship with God and was required to consecrate himself through various commands to be cleansed because of his sin. (See Leviticus 11:41–45.) His obedience to God's requirements for cleansing was a tangible sign of repentance, which was required under the Law to ensure their forgiveness and salvation. It was also necessary to obey God's commands in order to receive God's promises for health. (See Deuteronomy 7:11–15.)

Because we live under the provisions of the New Covenant, we receive forgiveness for our sins through faith in Christ because of His shed blood on the cross. Our repentance is expressed through a confession of faith in the sacrifice of Christ and followed by a surrender to follow Christ's commands. However, we are not made righteous by our good works, but through faith in Christ, who became our righteousness:

But of him are ye in Christ Jesus, who of God is made unto us wisdom, and righteousness, and sanctification, and redemption.

—1 Corinthians 1:30

Jesus Fulfilled the Mosaic Law

When Jesus said He came not to do away with the Law, but to fulfill it, He was validating the laws of the Old Testament. He was giving it His stamp of approval as the code of behavior by which we should live. Jesus did not tell us not to keep the moral laws. He raised a higher standard for the keeping of them.

Did Jesus ever tell us that we no longer need to follow the health and dietary laws of the Old Testament? No. It surprises many Christians to learn that Jesus actually kept all of these health laws Himself, and His disciples did also! As the last Prophet under the Old Covenant, Jesus kept all of the laws perfectly, something that no other human being on earth has done or will ever be able to do.

Because Jesus lived a sinless life as the Son of God, He was able to take our sins upon Himself on the cross. As He hung upon the tree and gasped out His final dying breath, His last words were, "It is finished" (John 19:30). He didn't only mean that His life on earth was through—He was declaring that the requirements of the Old Covenant had been fulfilled. By bearing our sins in His body, Christ had taken the brunt of God's wrath against sin for us.

No longer do we have to keep every single law in order to gain righteousness before God. The apostle Paul declared, "For Christ is the end of the law for righteousness to everyone who believes" (Rom. 10:4, NKJV). Jesus is now our righteousness, and when we place our faith in Him, we gain right standing with God, which establishes a new relationship with our heavenly Father.

Paul described this truth in the Book of Romans when he wrote that it is not by our works that we are saved, but by our faith. It is impossible for anyone to keep all of the Old Covenant laws perfectly—if it were up to our own abilities, we would surely be lost. But Paul also asked the question, "What shall we say then? Shall we continue in sin, that grace may abound?" (Rom. 6:1). Since Jesus has already died for us, and because doing good works is not what gets us into heaven, why should we keep the Law at all?

Jesus' work on the cross accomplished our righteousness so that our right standing with God is not contingent on our ability to keep the Law perfectly. However, if we choose to disobey God's laws, we will face consequences for which the Law was given to protect us. Christ's death did not undo the moral laws, making it acceptable to murder someone, tell a lie, commit adultery or steal. Neither did Christ's death change the composition of "unclean" foods, making it acceptable to eat as many fatty foods as we like, gain twenty extra pounds and risk damage to our bodies. One explicit New Testament situation affirms some of the dietary laws when outlining proper conduct for Gentile Christians:

*For it seemed good to the Holy Spirit, and to us, to lay upon you
no greater burden than these necessary things: that you abstain
from things offered to idols, from blood, from things strangled,
and from sexual immorality.*

—ACTS 15:28–29, NKJV

This passage at least shows that there was no precedent for abolishing
the dietary and health laws that had been a part of their lives under the
Mosaic Law. The apostle Paul clearly denounced doing anything that would
defile our bodies, which have become the temple of God. He declared:

*Know ye not that ye are the temple of God, and that the Spirit
of God dwelleth in you? If any man defile the temple of God,
him shall God destroy; for the temple of God is holy, which
temple ye are.*

—1 CORINTHIANS 3:16–17

The ancient Israelites would never have dreamed of desecrating God's
holy temple in their day; how much more should we obediently care for
our own bodies in which God Himself dwells?

Blessings and Consequences

If we choose to disobey God's commandments concerning our moral
behavior, there are consequences that no believer would question. If Joe mur-
ders his neighbor, even if Joe has a change of heart and accepts Christ as his
Savior, we still expect him to be sent to prison and face the consequences of
his actions. When a person lies, steals, becomes jealous or otherwise behaves
immorally, his actions bring consequences: Other people are hurt, lives are
ruined, and Satan has a field day for doing what he loves to do—kill, steal
and destroy (John 10:10). Much of the New Testament is dedicated to
teaching us how to walk in the love of God through obedience to these commandments. And these same Scriptures teach us there will always be consequences for disobeying God's moral laws.

In much the same way, if you choose to ignore God's laws regarding
your diet and your health, you open the door to the enemy to wreak havoc
in your life. Though God is not poised, waiting to pour out His wrath on
His children when they sin, the fact is you place yourself in harm's way
when you don't eat right or take care of your body properly. While you may
not have to sacrifice a sheep or a goat in the temple to restore your relationship with God, there are still unfortunate consequences of your actions:

- ❧ The Spirit of God is grieved. Because the Holy Spirit lives inside of you, He is grieved when you sin or do something to defile the temple of God—your body.

- ❧ You experience a loss of the fruit of the Spirit in your life.

- ❧ You open a door to the works of the enemy. Your failure to eat right may not cause you to lose your salvation, but it certainly can affect your health. The devil would love to take advantage of your poor choices to place sickness and disease on you and your family.

- ❧ You may be unable to fulfill God's destiny for your life and obey His command to be the light of the world. When you are sick in bed or too exhausted to move, you cannot be an effective witness for God.

One mistaken belief some people hold is that sin in a Christian's life somehow directly brings sickness to them, as if sickness were a punishment from God for our sin. What a sad and mistaken belief! It is our own poor choices that bring consequences to our lives in the form of sickness, which Christ died to heal. Though there are instances when choices have been made by people or generations before us that affect us, as in the case of innocent children who suffer disease, we still cannot fault a loving God for that tragedy.

An example of this mistaken belief is seen in the "plague" of AIDS, which some Christians believe was poured out by God to punish homosexuals for their sins. That is simply not true. God never desired that one homosexual—or anyone else—would die of AIDS. It is the behavior patterns that some people choose to practice, violating the laws of God, which place them at risk of disease. Unfortunately, many lives have been stolen because of AIDS. Obeying God's law for sexual relations would have prevented the consequences of contracting this dread plague. However, AIDS—or any other disease for that matter—did not come from God.

Jesus declared that He came to reveal the Father to us. His loving nature, reflected in His healing power to the multitudes, is a reflection of the Father's love. Jesus declared also that He came to bring us life and life more abundantly (John 10:10).

I have briefly discussed the relevance for Christians of the Bible's dietary and health laws because many of the Bible's health secrets presented in the

chapters of this book have their basis in these laws. I do not believe that
Scripture eliminates their relevance for today. And it is a scientific reality
that research is confirming their validity for our health and well-being in
today's culture. I encourage you to consider making them a part of your
life. As you do, I believe you will allow God to pour out His blessings of
health and restoration into your body, soul and spirit.

ASK DR. CHERRY

QUESTION: **What are the health benefits of following the
Old Testament prohibitions against eating fat?**

ANSWER: The Torah—the first five books of the Old Testament—
forbids the consumption of foods containing harmful fats (such as
LDL saturated fats):

> *It shall be a perpetual statute for your generations throughout all
> your dwellings, that ye eat neither fat nor blood.*
>   —LEVITICUS 3:17

> *Speak unto the children of Israel, saying, Ye shall eat no manner
> of fat, of ox, or of sheep, or of goat.*
>   —LEVITICUS 7:23

This prohibition against fat is especially important in our day. Over 50
percent of people in large industrialized countries die of heart disease,
which is most commonly caused by fat deposits building up in the
arteries, often starting as early in life as the teenage years. Many other
diseases are caused or exacerbated by the consumption of these LDL
(bad) saturated fats also.

To reduce your fat intake according to the Bible's standards and for
your own benefit:

- ꙮ Eat lean beef no more than three or four times a
  month.

- ꙮ Cook only with olive or canola oil.

- ꙮ Eat no meat at all three days per week. On those
  days, stick strictly to fruits and vegetables.

ᴄᴡ Eat fish at least two or three times a week, prefer-
ably "cold-water" fish (salmon, cod or herring)
because these are the fish that contain the beneficial omega-3 fatty acids.

Q UESTION: **According to the Bible, which animals are considered "clean" or "unclean"?**

A NSWER: The lists of clean and unclean animals found in Leviticus
11 and Deuteronomy 14 have important meaning for our lives today.
They are not a catalog of food taboos compiled at God's whim; they
demonstrate God's protection of His people and reflect a scientific reality
that was unheard of at that time: Animals can carry disease.

There are five general groups of animals listed in the Torah:

1. *Mammals*: The clean, furred animals belong to one type only,
   whether domesticated or wild. They are known as *ruminants*,
   or animals that chew the cud, and are some of our most
   important meat-producers. The simple rules for determining
   which mammal is "clean" is that it is to be both cloven-hoofed
   and a chewer of the cud. Those mammals that are one or the
   other are ruled unclean, such as the ones named: the camel,
   the coney, the hare and the pig (or swine) (Lev. 11:4–8). The
   pig is now known to host several serious parasites that are
   dangerous when ingested by humans. The pig is also considered a scavenger and may spread other diseases simply
   through contact with the animal. Eating pork is not safe unless
   it is thoroughly cooked, and then only in small quantities.

2. *Birds*: So many forms of birds exist that they cannot be
   specifically classified. Forbidden birds are named in
   Scripture: birds of prey, crows, buzzards and other carnivo-
   rous birds (Lev. 11:13–20). All other birds may be eaten.

3. *Reptiles*: Scripture says that "every creeping thing" that goes
   on its belly is forbidden for food (Lev. 11:42).

4. *Water animals*: Fish are not specifically named in any list, but
   they are included in the phrase "all that are in the waters"

(Lev. 11:9). Clean foods in this category must have fins and scales; thus all crustaceans, shellfish and the like are to be excluded from the diet.

5. *Insects*: The grasshopper, locust, cricket and katydid are the only clean insects listed in the Mosaic Law (Lev. 11:22, NIV). They are a useful food because of their high protein and caloric content. It is interesting to note that despite the vast numbers of insects on the earth, few types are actually eaten by any culture, even in countries short of animal protein.

Amazingly, the Bible lists foods that are acceptable for the health of our bodies as well as those that carry potentially unhealthy attributes that would be a risk to our health centuries before scientists discovered the reality of those potentials. Now it is common knowledge that pork can carry the deadly trichinosis infection and that shrimp and shellfish retain heavy metals such as mercury and lead, which are harmful to the human body. These are only examples of scientific knowledge that prove to us that God knows all things and that we can trust Him to know what is best for us!

CHAPTER 3

THE FAITH & MEDICINE CONNECTION

*He who does not use his endeavors to heal himself is
brother to him who commits suicide.*
—PROVERBS 18:9, AMP

C AN I GO TO A DOCTOR AND STILL WALK IN FAITH?" Many Christians
live under the misunderstanding that faith and medicine are sepa-
rate approaches to healing that contradict one another. It is wonderful to
enjoy the fresh revelation in the church today regarding divine healing
and faith. God is bringing healing to His people through this understanding of supernatural, instantaneous freedom from disease that is possible through faith.

However, in the midst of this incredible, healing move of God, there are
those among us who haven't received that instant miracle and who begin
to wonder, *Why haven't I been healed in this miraculous way?* They may
believe they have received a touch from God, sensing His presence in a
special way, but the symptoms of their disease remain. They may have
even received a supernatural healing, only to discover that the illness has
returned a few days or weeks later.

What should these people do? Are they exhibiting a "lack of faith" if
they decide to seek the advice of a physician? Why doesn't God heal them

22

miraculously as He does others? This is a dilemma with which many in the body of Christ grapple. Somehow we have the idea that the correct way for Christians to handle disease is to stand in faith, refusing medicine or other "natural" cures, and wait for a miracle. Divine healing is seen as the better solution to disease. Unfortunately, some people are so committed to this viewpoint that they may wait until their deathbed for their miraculous cure, and it still doesn't come. The inevitable results are devastating: A life that could have been lived out in fullness and health is cut short, and faith and trust in God are weakened, both in the patient and in the hearts of those around him or her.

"Do You Brush Your Teeth?"

When people wonder if they should "stand in faith" for their healing rather than seek a natural or medical solution, I like to ask them a very simple question: "Do you brush your teeth?" Of course, we all brush our teeth. But the next questions I ask are more important: "Don't you believe God can heal you of cavities? Can't He prevent plaque buildup and tooth decay from taking place? If so, why do you keep brushing your teeth?"

It's the same reasoning that keeps us from standing in front of a speeding train, raising our arms to heaven and expecting God to miraculously prevent us from getting hurt. My friends, disease can be heading your way; you may be right in its path. Wouldn't it make sense to do something simple—something natural—to prevent it from hitting you at full force? The Bible tells us:

> *He who does not use his endeavors to heal himself is brother to*
> *him who commits suicide.*
> —PROVERBS 18:9, AMP

I believe this verse can be interpreted to mean that we must do what we know to do to bring healing to our body, and then trust God for the rest. There is no validity to the faulty reasoning that concludes our healing must come either from God or from medical intervention. While we must learn to face every situation in faith, we cannot biblically support the claim that walking in faith excludes receiving the natural sources of healing God provided for us on this earth.

The Five P's of Spiritual Healing

There are five basic concepts—the key words of which begin with the letter *P*—that can help people determine what to do, both in the natural and in the spiritual realm, to receive the manifestation of their healing:

1. Understand that Jesus is the Great *Physician.* He is the One to whom you should turn first in times of trouble. He bore stripes on His back that you might be healed (1 Pet. 2:24). Look to Him for your answer.

2. Follow the *peace* of God. Don't pray out of fear or worry. You may not understand what's happening to you in the natural, but you can have God's peace in times of trouble. The Scriptures teach us to cast our cares upon the Lord (1 Pet. 5:7). The tense of this text implies that it is a continual process: Cast once, and then keep on casting!

3. Determine God's *pathway* to healing for you. Don't put God in a box or try to manipulate Him into doing what you want Him to do or healing you the way you think He should. If you ask, He will show you His plan for you, which will not be the same as one He showed to someone else.

4. Believe in the *power* of healing. When all else fails, stand! Stand in your faith and in your trust in God. Believe that He wants to heal you—that your healing has already been purchased on the cross—without limiting His method for healing you.

5. Pursue your healing with *persistence.* Hang in there. Jesus told parables to emphasize the importance of persevering in prayer, such as the widow who prevailed with the unjust judge (Luke 18:1–6).

God's Ways Are Not Our Ways

Why are some people miraculously healed while others are seemingly left to deal with their illnesses "on their own"? At first glance, this question seems to call into account the fairness of God. But the truth of the matter is that God loves each of us completely—no more or no less than another—and His desire to heal is unlimited. He is a holy and just God. But He chooses to deal with each of His children in different ways.

One person may indeed receive a miraculous and instantaneous healing from diabetes when prayed for in a healing crusade, while another who is stricken with diabetes may find that the pathway to healing includes diet, exercise and even medication to keep the diabetes under control. Both persons will experience health and longevity in their lives, but God, in His wisdom, chose different paths for them to take to get to that place of healing.

Earlier in this book I mentioned Jesus healing a blind man by placing a mixture of mud and saliva on the man's eyes and then giving further instructions for the man to go wash in the Pool of Siloam to receive his healing (John 9). However, on another occasion, Jesus healed two blind men by simply touching their eyes and commanding them to see (Matt. 20:29–34). He healed blind Bartimaeus by simply saying, "Go thy way; thy faith hath made thee whole" (Mark 10:46–52.)

Now, if we are honest with ourselves, most of us would admit that we would rather be healed the way Bartimaeus was healed. Not only does it seem easier, but also it might give us a more exciting story to tell! The fact is, however, that all four blind men were healed—they could see. The only difference was that the blind man whose story is recorded in John 9 was allowed to participate in the process of his healing. Jesus required certain acts of obedience from him in order to receive healing.

It is a common misconception that it takes much more faith to be healed instantly and supernaturally of a disease than to seek healing with the help of a physician. And many wrongly believe that if a person has to seek a physician for help in dealing with the symptoms of a disease, his or her faith has failed. But really, is it harder or easier to trust God when you see immediate results? I believe it sometimes requires greater faith for us to walk through an illness and seek God's face to find our pathway to healing than it does to receive an instant, miraculous healing from God. We have only to look at the Bible heroes in the Scriptures to know that our faith was meant to take us *through* some difficult situations, not just to keep us *from* them.

Healing Anointing Flows Through Natural Substances

The minute Jesus touched the two blind men in Matthew 20 and the blind man in John 9, His anointing was released into them to effect their healing. They suffered from the same disease—blindness—and in the end, their healings were exactly the same—they could see. But the paths they took to get there were quite different.

When Jesus created the mixture of mud and saliva, it became an anointed salve for the blind man's eyes. Note that the mixture was made of natural things of this earth—mud and saliva. In that sense, it is not unlike many medications and treatments we use today; they are natural, made from the earth and within the realm of man's understanding. However, when Jesus touched that natural mixture of mud and saliva, He anointed it with His healing power. Then He gave the man instructions to go and wash in the Pool of Siloam.

God's pathway to healing will always involve an element of faith to receive His healing power through spiritual or natural means. And it will include instructions that are specifically tailored to the individual. He knows what each person needs and what will most effectively bring about that person's total healing.

Many suggestions in this book are natural remedies that can often provide better results than traditional medicine—and *with less or no side effects!* It may surprise you to know that even 40 to 50 percent of all prescription medications are derived from God's natural plant kingdom. They are His provision for our healing, as suggested by Scripture:

> *The leaves of the tree were for the healing of the nations.*
> —Revelation 22:2, nkjv

A Proper Perspective

As a Christian physician, I cannot view medicine and faith as contradictory issues. Healing received by faith or through medical intervention is not an "either, or" issue. When a Christian comes to me seeking help with an ailment or disease, I do not consider that his faith has failed. Instead, I consider that through the medical knowledge we gain through diagnosis, we have important tools to help us target our prayers against the specific enemy that has brought disease to the patient's body. Such knowledge helps the patient and me find the pathway to healing that God ordains for him or her. All knowledge comes from God, and He has instructed us to acknowledge Him in all of our ways so that He can direct our paths (Prov. 3:6).

The most important key to finding a solution to your illness is to seek God's pathway to healing for *you*—the set of instructions that He has specifically ordained for you to follow that will ultimately set you free from the effects of disease. Chances are, it will not be the same pathway as the one God has for your friend, your neighbor or even another family member. He has a plan specifically suited for you and you alone. You have been fearfully and wonderfully made (Ps. 139)! There is no other creature like you, and your Creator knows exactly what to do to heal your body.

❧ ASK DR. CHERRY

QUESTION: **When I am sick, whom should I call, my pastor or my doctor?**

ANSWER: Call both! There doesn't have to be a conflict of interest between the two. Consult a doctor to find out exactly what the situation is with which you are dealing, and then call your pastor with the specifics so that he will know exactly how to pray.

QUESTION: **Should I have more tests done, or should I simply stand in faith for my healing?**

ANSWER: Many tests that doctors perform can help in determining the cause and/or scope of a disease. The information that medical tests provide can empower your prayers against the illness because they provide specifics against which you can target your prayers. However, some tests can also be difficult or uncomfortable to undergo, so the first prayer you should pray is that you know which tests to undergo.

A comforting verse of Scripture declares, "And let the peace of God rule in your hearts [as an umpire]" (Col. 3:15). Begin to ask God to give you His peace when you pray about certain tests that you are facing. If you feel a continual sense of anxiety or dread every time you think or pray about a certain procedure, that may not be the path God would have you take. But if His peace begins to flood your heart about a certain test or procedure, you can be assured that the divine "umpire" is ruling in your heart, indicating what the right course of action is for you to take.

QUESTION: **Is alternative medicine an acceptable choice for Christians to use?**

ANSWER: Many alternative types of medicine—such as vitamin therapy or acupuncture—are becoming more popular in America today. Whether you should choose to pursue them is a decision that should be made after much prayer. The Holy Spirit guides us into all truth, and He will show you the right path for your healing.

QUESTION: **What should I do when I am hospitalized for an illness?**

ANSWER: Being in the hospital can be a frightening and often confusing experience. First of all, it is important to resolve the misconception that being in the hospital is contradictory to walking in faith as a believer. Sometimes medical intervention is a necessary step in the healing process. God's presence goes with you into the hospital just as He goes with you everywhere else. You can exercise your faith in a hospital bed as effectively as you can at home.

What many patients fail to realize is that information is key to making right decisions for their health. Ask your doctor questions. Be sure you understand what courses of treatment are available to you and what the effects—both pro and con—are for each possible treatment. Becoming as informed as possible about your disease will help you feel more comfortable in making decisions, and you will know better how to pray.

Sometimes patients have trouble determining when their doctor will make his rounds in the hospital so that they can be prepared to ask him the questions they need answered. One suggestion I have given is to call the doctor's office (perhaps early in the morning when they begin to answer their phones) and ask what time he will be visiting your particular hospital on that day. Make a list of questions to ask him so that nothing important is forgotten.

Finally, remember that the doctor will always present you with the worst-case scenario. That's his job. Instead of thinking of him as the bearer of bad news, begin to view him as a messenger of God sent to tell you the truth, to show you how to pray and to give you the options you need to understand in order to discover your pathway to healing. An original definition of a physician was a teacher. We need to think of our doctors in that way: They are teachers sent by God to show us the things that we can do in the natural to help prevent or treat a condition. And the knowledge they give us will help us to know more specifically how to pray.

CHAPTER 4

THE BIBLE'S ULTIMATE HEALTH SECRET

The effective, fervent prayer of
a righteous man avails much.
—JAMES 5:16, NKJV

P RAYER IS A POTENT WEAPON AGAINST DISEASE. Many patients and doctors today are frustrated by their inability to effectively prevent or halt the progression of disease. Even with all of the technological advances in medicine and healthcare in the last several decades, mankind has not been able to eradicate the presence of illness. Even the common cold is still prevalent, not to mention the major killers stalking us—cardiovascular disease, cancer and diabetes, just to name a few.

The Effective Weapon of Prayer

In the face of these overwhelming odds, what are we to do? As a Christian physician, I can tell you that my primary weapon against disease is prayer. When I see patients who are ravaged by the effects of a particular illness, or what is worse, their test results and case history are inconclusive so that we are not sure what is causing the symptoms, I do not turn first to further testing or to my prescription pad. I turn to what I consider to be the

Bible's greatest health secret: the effective weapon of prayer.

Doctors are only human, and the medical community has limited options. What are you to do when a doctor has done everything he knows to do, tried every treatment available and prescribed every possible medication, but still you do not improve?

Many people who are adrift in the world without God or His Word begin to lose hope and to despair that they will ever recover. But as a Christian, you need never lose hope. You should always turn to the almighty God, the One who created your body and who knows how to fix it. He created this world and all of the natural remedies available in it, and He sent His Son to purchase your healing with His very blood. This powerful, loving God is on your side! And when you turn to Him, He will always be with you and give you the answer to your deepest needs. The apostle Paul declared this wonderful reality:

> *For I am persuaded, that neither death, nor life, nor angels, nor principalities, nor powers, nor things present, nor things to come, nor height, nor depth, nor any other creature, shall be able to separate us from the love of God, which is in Christ Jesus our Lord.*
> —ROMANS 8:38–39

"I Don't Know How to Pray"

Everyone will face a moment of crisis, a midnight hour, at some point in his or her life. For some, the moment comes sooner than for others, but rest assured, your moment will come. What will happen at that time? Will you know what to do? Will you know how to pray?

When many of my patients are faced with serious health crises, they don't know what to do or how to pray effectively. They haven't been prepared for this dark moment. Fortunately, God in His wisdom and providence has given us in His Word the answers we need for all of life's situations. When my patients ask me to help them pray, I happily show them what the Bible teaches.

In fact, Jesus' disciples asked Him the very question that my patients ask me. They had seen their Master's prayer life—the many times that He would retreat to be alone with His Father and pray, sometimes all night—and they saw the power and effectiveness with which He healed the masses. For that reason, they came to Him one day, entreating Him, "Lord, teach us to pray" (Luke 11:1). Jesus provided them with the pattern prayer that we still use today, the prayer called the "Lord's Prayer."

I believe that Jesus gave this prayer to the disciples—and to us today—not only for us to memorize and recite, but also to teach us the basic principles involved in praying. This simple prayer embodies certain fundamentals that we should understand and apply to all our prayers. As we focus briefly on these important aspects of effective prayer, I encourage you to begin to use them in your prayers with renewed faith.

"Our Father which art in heaven, Hallowed be thy name" (Matt. 6:9). We must begin our prayer by acknowledging God as our Father. In His great love, He is our Provider, the One who knows us and knows what we need and what is best for us. He is interested in our welfare and is lovingly approachable to His children at any time.

"Thy kingdom come. Thy will be done in earth, as it is in heaven" (v. 10). As the ultimate "higher power," God's kingdom supercedes—and overrides—all earthly governments. As we learn to recognize that His will is always good, we seek to follow Him always and desire His direction of our lives.

"Give us this day our daily bread" (v. 11). God is the Source for everything we need in our lives on a daily basis. We should ask Him specifically to provide for our needs—including health and healing for every part of our being.

"And forgive us our debts [transgressions, trespasses], *as we forgive our debtors"* (v. 12). God's perfection can obliterate our imperfections, His wisdom far exceeds ours, and His divine mercy and grace are able to save to the uttermost when we seek forgiveness for our sins. It is important to remember that we are forgiven when we forgive others. (See Matthew 6:14–15.)

"And lead us not into temptation, but deliver us from evil" (v. 13). There is evil as well as good in the world, and there are things that we may be tempted to do (such as smoking, drinking excessively, gluttonous eating habits) that could adversely affect our health and our ability to ward off disease. Only with God's active help that we entreat through prayer can we overcome the many pitfalls, problems, opposition and temptations that we will inevitably confront.

"For thine is the kingdom, and the power, and the glory, for ever. Amen" (v. 13). Our success in prayer, in our lives and in our health will depend on our understanding and remembering who God is, what He asks of us and how we cultivate relationship to Him.

With this guidance received from Jesus' example, it seems easier to understand how God wants you to pray. But how can you apply this type of prayer to those troubled and confusing times of illness and disease? Below I have listed five specific ways you can pray for your healing when you need it the most.

Five Ways to Pray for Your Healing

When you or a loved one is faced with a terrible disease, what is the first thing you should do? To whom should you turn? The psalmist declared, "God is our refuge and strength, a very present help in trouble" (Ps. 46:1). The psalms are filled with prayers and cries from people in desperate trouble who rejoiced when God heard their cries and delivered them. You may turn to their prayers and pray them in your hour of need as well, expecting your loving heavenly Father to answer you as well. But sometimes it is difficult to know exactly how to pray specifically in times of crises. Here are five effective ways I have found to pray when you are facing a health crisis.

1. Pray for openness to hear God's voice.

After a diagnosis, you may be overwhelmed with unsolicited advice from well-meaning friends or loved ones, or from someone who has faced a similar illness. You may also face confusing decisions as to which tests or procedures to undergo or which medical options to pursue. Your doctor may be biased toward a certain treatment option and may be pressuring you to make decisions for which you feel unprepared.

The first step to take at such a time is to pray for God's voice to cut through the din of all other voices and clearly make Himself and His will known. His way will provide the greatest peace and can direct you toward the most effective path for your healing.

2. Pray to know how to pray.

Sometimes the confusion can be so great that you may feel at a loss to know how to pray for your healing. The Holy Spirit is your heavenly guide—your instructor in the things of God (John 16:13). He is willing and available to show you how to pray. Begin to spend time waiting on God, and ask the Holy Spirit to give you the words to pray.

3. Pray for correct understanding of Scripture.

When you understand what God's Word has to say about health and healing, and God's role in that healing process, you will become more effective in your prayers. There are three major biblical truths about healing that you need to accept when seeking God for healing.

First, you must first understand that *God wants you to be healed!* Read the following scriptures, and allow them to sink deep into your heart, building your faith for healing:

～ "I am the LORD who heals you" (Exod. 15:26, NKJV).

~ "I will take sickness away from the midst of you" (Exod. 23:25, NKJV).

~ "And the LORD will take away from you all sickness" (Deut. 7:15, NKJV).

~ "He sent His word and healed them" (Ps. 107:20, NKJV).

~ "'I will restore health to you and heal you of your wounds,' says the LORD" (Jer. 30:17, NKJV).

~ "He...healed all who were sick" (Matt. 8:16, NKJV).

~ "They will lay hands on the sick, and they will recover" (Mark 16:18, NKJV).

~ "...by whose stripes you were healed" (1 Pet. 2:24, NKJV).

Second, agree to accept the biblical truth that *the price for your healing has already been paid*—by Jesus Christ on the cross! When Jesus came to earth, mankind faced not one, but two tremendous needs—he was hopelessly sinful in his heart, and his body desperately needed healing. Strange as it may seem, while all Christians believe that Christ died on the cross to redeem mankind from sin, some are not sure about God's provision for healing. They have never understood that on the same day Jesus was crucified, He also took upon Himself our sicknesses, providing redemption for the body of man as well as for his soul.

If we believe in salvation—through Christ's sacrifice on the cross to forgive our sins—then, according to the Scriptures, we must believe in physical healing as well. The Bible declares of Christ's death: "Himself took our infirmities, and bare our sicknesses" (Matt. 8:17). The terrible price Christ paid on Calvary bought our physical healing as well as our salvation from sin.

Third, the Bible teaches us to *persevere in prayer.* Too often, we expect to receive answers from God instantly, and if they do not appear immediately, we pout and say that God did not hear us. But, as we have mentioned, Jesus taught us to persevere in our prayer efforts. In Luke 18, He told a parable of an unjust judge to illustrate His point. The first verse of that chapter tells us, "And he spake a parable unto them to this end, that men ought always to pray, and not to faint." Then He told of a judge who neither feared God nor regarded man. When a widow came to him seeking for justice, he ignored her at first, but she kept coming back and crying out to him. Finally the judge said, "Though I fear not God, nor regard man; yet because this widow troubleth me, I will avenge her, lest by her continual coming she weary me" (Luke 18:4–5).

We must not think we are "twisting God's arm" to get an answer; He is not an unjust judge. The Scriptures are clear that we often wrestle against unseen enemies that do not give in easily in their desire to defeat us. (See Daniel 9; Ephesians 6.) Jesus' point was this: "And shall not God avenge his own elect, which cry day and night unto him, though he bear long with them? I tell you that he will avenge them speedily" (Luke 18:7–8). God places a high premium on developing perseverance in His children so that they can defeat the most stubborn enemy.

Have you prayed to be healed and the answer has not come? Pray again, and keep on praying. Don't give up. Be persistent. How often should you pray, and how long should you persevere? The Bible says, "Pray without ceasing" (1 Thess. 5:17). And again, "Praying always with all prayer and supplication in the Spirit, and watching thereunto with all perseverance..." (Eph. 6:18). Be patient. Be faithful. Be determined. Keep praying and believing, and persevere until the answer comes.

4. Specifically target your prayers against your disease.

Become informed about your illness. Learn as many specifics as you can. This is where your doctor can help. Arm yourself against the enemy with as much information as you can gather, and then actively pray, using that information to your advantage. For instance, if your doctor tells you that a specific artery near your heart is becoming blocked and causing cardiovascular difficulties, then pray specifically for that particular artery, that it would become clear, in the name of Jesus! Or if there is a cancerous growth in your body, find out specifically where it is, and then continually lay your hands on that part of your body, commanding the cancer to shrink and disappear.

5. Pray for your own individual pathway to healing.

Perhaps most importantly, pray for God to make clear His pathway to healing—the path that He has designed specifically for you. Use the knowledge from your doctor and from advice given in later chapters of this book to direct you. Bring the options that your doctor presents to you before the throne of grace, and ask the Father which way He would have you to go. Remember, God wants you to be healed! As you acknowledge Him, He will give you His peace and will guide you with His Holy Spirit into the way you should go.

ASK DR. CHERRY

QUESTION: **How can I know if my doctor is following the best course of treatment for me?**

ANSWER: Pray about all of the treatment options that are available to you. As I mentioned earlier, Colossians 3:15 tells us that the peace of God will guard your heart and mind when you are following what God tells you to do. The Amplified Version reads that His peace will "rule [act as umpire continually]" in your heart. That divine Umpire has the final word! Pray for the peace of God to rest upon the treatment option that is right for you. I suggest you pray for turmoil of heart and mind to signal that you are turning in the wrong direction. Ask the Father to make clear which way you are to go, and then, with His peace, be obedient to follow what He tells you.

QUESTION: **What do I do if I don't see my prayers answered right away?**

ANSWER: Most pathways of healing will not bring instantaneous results. God will often take you through a *process* of healing during which He works His redemptive plan for your body, your mind and your heart. As you look to Him, He fills your heart with faith, transforms your character to be more like Christ and allows you to participate in the healing process through believing prayer. This process will help you to learn to trust God more completely as your Father and your Healer. Once you have determined what you know God wants you to do, continue to follow your pathway to healing with patience and perseverance.

NATURAL HEALTH
SECRETS FOR
CURING DISEASE

CHAPTER 5

BEATING HEART DISEASE

My son, do not forget my law, but let your heart keep my commands; for length of days and long life and peace they will add to you.
—PROVERBS 3:1–2, NKJV

HEART DISEASE IS A KILLER. Have you ever heard of someone dying of a heart attack who was the least likely person you would expect to suffer heart disease? Seemingly healthy people in their prime—including football stars and other athletes—fall over dead, sometimes even after just having passed a physical at their doctor's office. Contrary to what it might look like on the surface, the heart attack did not take place as suddenly as it seemed. More than likely, underlying problems had remained undetected and untreated in that person's body—perhaps for years—that eventually killed him or her.

You may be aware that the cardiovascular system is the system in your body that circulates blood, carrying life-giving oxygen *to* and poisonous waste products *from* your vital organs. The word *cardiovascular* means "pertaining to the heart and the blood vessels." Therefore, *cardiovascular disease* is any disease that would affect those areas of the body.

Cardiovascular disease is the number one killer today—even among Christians—often striking suddenly and without warning. One in every two Americans dies of cardiovascular disease. (That's *50 percent!*) Heart disease kills twice as many people as all forms of cancer combined.[1] This crisis affects us all, whether we are facing it in our own bodies or watching it happen to someone we love. But the good news is that it is possible to prevent and even reverse cardiovascular disease before it becomes deadly.

Although our archenemy Satan, whose purpose is to kill, steal and destroy (John 10:10), would like to wipe out as many people in the body of Christ as possible through heart or vascular illness, God has provided everything that our bodies need to counteract this deadly killer. Our first step is to educate ourselves about our bodies and how they function, and then learn the methods and substances that God would have us use to restore and maintain our body's health.

As you will see in this chapter, cardiovascular disease involves more than just heart attacks. It encompasses a host of ailments that affect the heart, blood vessels, veins and arteries. We will examine the most common of these ailments, which may be affecting your health without your even being aware of them. How much do you know about your heart?

Anatomy of the Heart

The human heart is a strong muscle, used to pump blood through the arteries and veins, dispensing important nutrients and oxygen and carrying waste material away from the cells. There are four chambers in the heart. The two upper chambers—the atria—are smaller than the two lower chambers—the ventricles—the large pumping chambers that propel the blood out of the heart and throughout the body. The right ventricle pumps blood to the lungs; the left ventricle pumps blood to the rest of the body.

Arrhythmia: Irregular heartbeats

Most people who experience arrhythmia don't go in to see their doctor and say, "I've got an irregular heartbeat, Doc. I think I might have an arrhythmia." Many people aren't even aware that they are experiencing an arrhythmia. Their observations may be something like, "My heart has been doing flip-flops lately," or, "I've been having palpitations." Sometimes they may feel as if their heart has paused or skipped a beat, which can be quite frightening to people who don't understand what is happening to them. Some people may even begin to wonder if they are about to have a heart attack. If their heartbeat pauses for longer than a beat, they wonder if their heart will start to beat again!

Arrhythmia, or irregular heartbeat, is a very common condition. In fact, all of us have a type of irregular heartbeat called a *sinus arrhythmia,* which is actually quite normal. If you were to be sitting in your chair, resting and breathing at a normal pace, and you happened to take your pulse at that time, you might notice that your pulse was not occurring at an entirely steady rate. It may speed up slightly and then just slow back down. Heart rates often vary according to a person's breathing pattern or other changes that are occurring in the body. Becoming aware that this is a normal occurrence will keep you from feeling alarmed.

A study was done on a group of medical students during which each of them was hooked up to an electrocardiogram that measured their resting heart rates. Even though these were young, healthy, college-age students, every single one of them—that's *100 percent*—had irregularities in their heart rhythms. Most students were completely unaware of their arrhythmia, and almost all of the irregularities were benign.[2]

Sinus arrhythmia is nothing at all about which to be alarmed. In fact, it is a good idea for you to become aware of the usual heart rate patterns that occur in your own body so that you can detect the more dangerous forms of arrhythmia that could occur in case of disease.

Bradycardia

One heart irregularity to which we must pay much closer attention is *bradycardia.* The root word for *brady* means "slow," and *cardia,* of course, refers to the heart; therefore, bradycardia indicates that a person's heart is beating more slowly than it should.

The immediate question that probably comes to your mind is, *How do I know how slow is too slow?* First of all, as I have stated, it is important for you to get to know your own body. Many athletes who are in peak physical condition will have slower heart rates than people who are not in shape. I am a runner, and because I run on a regular basis, my own heart rate is lower than that of many people. But on the average, if your resting heart rate drops to fifty beats per minute or lower, you could be experiencing bradycardia. If that is the case, you should get your heart rate checked by your doctor.

God placed within your heart a natural defense against bradycardia. A misfiring of the electrical impulses of the heart, which could cause bradycardia, is controlled by the *sinoatrial node,* a "natural pacemaker." When it triggers a conduction pathway, electricity passes through the A-V node (atrioventricular node) of the heart tissue, which in turn causes the lower ventricles of the heart to contract and pump blood. When everything is functioning normally, the sinus node fires regularly, usually around seventy to seventy-five beats per minute. But if there is a problem, perhaps some scar tissue or other disruption of the electrical impulse, the ventricles do not receive the signal to contract. At that point, your heart would conceivably stop beating and you would be in serious trouble, except for God's wonderful protective design.

God designed your heart to keep beating even if there is a disruption of the electrical signals; the ventricles will contract on their own, continuing to send life-giving blood to your brain and other vital organs. It is a survival mechanism, designed to keep you alive. The problem is that the contractions will only occur at about forty beats per minute. At that rate, you will notice that something is very wrong. Because there isn't enough blood circulating, you will become light-headed, dizzy, perhaps even disoriented. When this happens, it is time to seek medical attention. Bradycardia—slow heartbeat—can signal that there is a problem with this built-in pacemaker that God designed. If it is not kicking in correctly, your heart rate can drop dangerously low, and your vital organs—especially the brain—can experience a devastating lack of blood flow.

What can be done to correct this potentially dangerous situation? First of all, as I mentioned earlier, accurate, specific knowledge about what is wrong is helpful to let you know how to target your prayers. You can begin to pray specifically for the sinus node, that it would function normally and that the nerve impulses it sends would flow correctly through the heart and cause it to pump blood in the way that it should. A medical answer for people whose built-in pacemakers are not functioning correctly sometimes involves inserting a surgically implanted pacemaker into the heart to keep it beating regularly.

There are more causes of bradycardia than the misfiring of the electrical impulses in the heart. An abnormally low heart rate can also be an indication of a thyroid problem. Because the thyroid gland is the master gland that controls metabolism in the body—including heart rate—if the hormones from the thyroid are not at the correct level, your heart rate can slow down. Your doctor can order a simple test called an *Ultra-sensitive T.S.H.* that will test your thyroid hormone levels to rule out this problem.

Tachycardia

At the opposite extreme from bradycardia is the condition of *tachycardia,* meaning a heart rate that is too rapid. The prefix *tachy* means "fast," and, again, *cardia* means "heart." Tachycardia is generally defined as a resting heart rate that is over one hundred beats per minute.

Tachycardia can be caused by a variety of conditions. One of the first things that doctors will check for is anemia, or a low blood count. Some people with anemia will experience heart rates of up to one hundred twenty beats per minute. If you have a drop in your hemoglobin, which carries oxygen to your tissues and organs, you will start to experience a lack of oxygen in those tissues. God has designed the body to signal the heart to beat faster when this occurs so that more blood will be carried throughout the body in a shorter period of time. We truly are fearfully and wonderfully made! If you are experiencing an unusually high heart rate, ask your doctor to perform a simple blood test (CBC) to determine whether or not you are anemic. It can tell you the levels of iron in your blood, the number of red blood cells and so on; the CBC can also help point to a solution to your heart rate problem.

Tachycardia can also be a symptom of an underlying infection somewhere in the body. On the average, for every degree of above-normal temperature (fever) in the body, the heart rate goes up ten beats per minute. So if your heart begins to beat faster on a consistent basis, begin to ask God to show you if there are any infections lurking in your body of which you might be unaware. Have your doctor perform a check of your white blood cell count to see if your body is under attack. Perhaps your immune system has been weakened by poor nutrition or some other reason. A weakened immune system can be strengthened by increasing appropriate supplement support that will help your body fight off infection.

Premature supraventricular tachycardia

Another type of arrhythmia, called *premature supraventricular tachycardia (PSVT),* can be as frightening as it sounds! Most arrhythmias cause you to feel as though your heart has just done a flip-flop or even skipped a beat or two; those are usually premature contractions of the atria, the upper chambers of the heart, and are generally benign. However, when PSVT occurs, you could be calmly sitting in an easy chair, breathing normally, when suddenly your heart takes off on a full-speed gallop, sometimes reaching a rate of two hundred twenty beats per minute. That's enough to get anyone's attention!

Many people rush to the emergency room, convinced they are having a heart attack. However, what has happened is that the upper chambers of the heart begin to beat on their own at a super rate of speed. The lower chambers are not beating fast enough to keep up, so they begin to fill poorly with blood, causing you to feel nauseated, light-headed or dizzy. Sometimes the problem lasts only a few seconds and then goes away, but it can last up to eight or ten hours, which is what usually causes a person to panic.

The enemy loves to plant fear in our hearts, and he is especially effective when he uses deceit to do so. The fact is that PSVT is usually a harmless phenomenon. Even in the emergency room, one of the age-old treatments that doctors will use to treat it is one of the simplest: breathing into a paper bag. By doing so, the levels of carbon dioxide in your bloodstream are raised, which terminates the irregular heart rhythm. Some other tricks that are also effective include coughing as hard as possible, holding your breath for twenty seconds or splashing cold water in the face. These simple treatments cause enough of a shock to your system that your heart rate is brought back to normal.

Isn't it amazing how something so frightening can be remedied by such simple methods? Many doctors' first response is to take out a prescription pad and give you a pill or two to take. But wouldn't a better approach to the problem be offering the patient a paper bag to breathe into, which could solve the problem simply? Paper bags don't have side effects! A good principle to follow is to try the simple solutions first before reaching for a pill or medication that could cause you further problems.

Atrial fibrillation

A more dangerous form of irregular heartbeat is called *atrial fibrillation*. The term *atrial* refers to the upper chambers of the heart, and *fibrillation* means "a shaking or a quivering motion." Therefore, atrial fibrillation is a quivering that occurs in the upper chambers of the heart. A good comparison to what goes on would be that of the agitator in the washing machine that slaps the clothes around in the water to get them clean. However, when the atria of the heart begin to agitate in this manner, they aren't stirring up soap and water; they're affecting platelets that are in the bloodstream. When these platelets are stimulated in such a manner, they begin to stick together, forming the dangerous condition of a blood clot. The blood clot then finds its way into the ventricles of the heart, where it can be pumped into the carotid or vertebral arteries, go straight to the brain and cause a stroke.

Because atrial fibrillation can cause such a dangerous situation, it is important to have a checkup performed occasionally. Most people suffering from atrial fibrillation would not be able to feel it occurring in their chest. If the condition is diagnosed, there are several ways to treat it. The first course of action is to prevent the platelets in the blood from sticking together. For younger people (under the age of seventy), a simple dose of aspirin (325 milligrams per day) is effective. However, if a person is over the age of seventy, a blood thinner is usually required.

If you are using a blood thinner, you will need to have your blood monitored through tests to adjust the dosage. If your blood becomes too thin, you will have a tendency to bleed, but if it is not thin enough, it will not be effective in blocking the formation of blood clots in the heart. Interestingly, if the blood clot tendency is prevented, even if the atrial fibrillation is not brought under control, the condition is usually no longer a health issue.

Sometimes atrial fibrillation can indicate a problem in one of the valves in the heart. I recommend that you ask your doctor to perform an echocardiogram to check for this condition. (He probably will anyway.) If a valve is too narrow or has developed stenosis (thickening), the blood may not be passing through it correctly and may be disrupting the beating of the heart.

If you are experiencing atrial fibrillation, arm yourself with the information you have just received and take it before the Lord in prayer. Begin to command your platelets, in the name of Jesus, to *not* clump themselves together or form blood clots in your heart. Speak to the atria of your heart and command them to beat regularly, in the manner that God intended for them to do. Seek the wisdom of the Father to know what pathway to take, whether it be a dose of aspirin or a regimen of blood thinners. Remember, He has a pathway to healing designed just for you.

Premature ventricular contraction

All of us will experience premature ventricular contractions (PVCs) at one time or another, but it is when they become a consistent pattern that they become very dangerous. In a normal heartbeat, just before the electrical impulse is fired, there is an instant of time called "repolarization." It occurs just after the completion of one heartbeat, during which the heart is preparing to beat again. However, if the heart fires off too early, there will then be a long pause, and the ventricles of the heart begin to overfill with blood. This causes the ventricles to stretch and then beat strongly to push all of the blood into the bloodstream. You will notice this strong heartbeat and will often have to pause for breath or cough in order to recover.

Many times premature ventricular contraction can be caused by stress, too much caffeine or even stimulants found in over-the-counter cold medicines (pseudoephedrines). Most of the time, the situation is benign. However, if there are three or more of this type of heartbeats that occur right in a row, something called *ventricular tachycardia,* or VT, occurs. When VT occurs, which involves several longer pauses in a row between heartbeats, there is no time for the heart to fill with blood. Suddenly there is a shortage of blood being pumped from the heart. People have been known to pass out at this point from the lack of circulation to their brains. Once this dangerous cycle has begun, the person may progress quickly from VT to a very serious problem called *ventricular fibrillation.*

You may be familiar with the term *ventricular fibrillation* from watching the television show *ER*. When the doctor shouts out, "He's going into VFIB!", this is the condition to which he is referring. Ventricular fibrillation is very different from atrial fibrillation because it affects the large pumping chambers of the heart. If these chambers begin to quiver, they are not pumping blood effectively, and the person will die very quickly if drastic measures—usually an electrical shock to the heart—are not taken. I encourage you to seek medical advice if you are aware of a pattern of symptoms we described, feeling strong heartbeats that take your breath, especially if they occur continually.

Natural Substances to Prevent or Reverse Arrhythmia

God has provided several natural substances that have proven to be very effective in the prevention and treatment of these cardiovascular problems we have just discussed. As you seek to approach your situation in the simplest way first, I suggest you consider the following supplements as valid options, along with prayer and seeking medical advice.

Coenzyme Q_{10}

Coenzyme Q_{10} has proven effective in stabilizing the normal rhythm of the heart, which is the primary cause of many forms of cardiovascular disease. A dosage of 50 milligrams per day will strengthen the heart muscle and allow it to beat with stability.

Magnesium

Right behind coenzyme Q_{10} in effectiveness against cardiovascular disease is magnesium. In fact, for years magnesium was used in hospital IVs to help stabilize patients' heart rates. Four hundred milligrams daily will stabilize the electrical disturbances in the heart.

Omega-3 fatty acids (fish oil)

There are many benefits to omega-3 oils, but one benefit that has been proven in medical journal studies is that omega-3 oils stabilize irregular heartbeats. You should take a dose of 2,000 milligrams per day.

Potassium

Potassium levels that are either too high or too low will frequently cause irregular heart rates. Generally, a dose of 99 milligrams daily of potassium is sufficient.

Calcium

There are four basic forms of calcium, and I always tell my patients to get their calcium from more than one form. *Carbonate* (found in Tums), while the most common form of calcium, is not the most easily absorbed. *Citrate* is the most absorbable form, but *lactate* (found in milk) and *ascorbate* are also available. Calcium has a double benefit: It can both stabilize heart rate and lower blood pressure. You should take 500 milligrams of calcium per day.

It is best to combine these supplements in your regimen because their effect is synergistic, meaning their effectiveness multiplies when they are used together.

The Real Causes of Heart Attacks

Two of the most frightening words that a person can hear are the words *heart attack.* That is understandable because of the history of tragedy heart attacks represent to lives and families. The good news is that there are new discoveries that are making it possible for us to prevent heart attacks—and to do so in a natural way.

As I mentioned in the beginning of this chapter, it is often a mystery why seemingly healthy people—even athletes—can just keel over and die of a heart attack without any warning whatsoever. In fact, many people who have had heart attacks report having never had a symptom before their first heart attack occurred. The answer to this mystery lies in an understanding of how buildup of plaque in the arteries actually takes place.

For years doctors had believed that an artery was like a water pipe, which slowly collected plaque over the years, causing a buildup that eventually blocked the artery and caused a heart attack. That is what I was taught in medical school, and it certainly seemed to be a logical explanation. Unfortunately, as we are just now starting to discover, it was wrong.

The arteries that are 90 percent blocked, we are learning, are *not* the arteries that cause most heart attacks! People with blocked arteries often experience *angina,* which is defined as chest pain on exertion. It is difficult for the blood to flow through their arteries when they exert themselves. But often in heart attacks, there is a sudden onset of chest pain, which begins in the middle of the chest and radiates outward, often through the left side and down the left arm.

What is happening is that fatty plaque develops not just within the artery itself, but also in the *wall* of the artery. This plaque, which is covered by the lining of the arterial wall, builds up and actually causes the lining of the artery to rupture. When that happens, suddenly, the fatty material within the wall begins to protrude into the blood flow in the artery.

Because our bodies were created to repair themselves, when they detect any breach, such as the arterial rupture, the body's healing process signals a blood clot to form. In this case, the effects of that natural healing process can be disastrous. Platelets begin to stick together, a clot begins to form, and in a period of a few minutes, that clot fills up the artery, blocking blood flow. In addition, the artery itself begins to constrict in order to stop the flow of blood from the breach in the wall's lining—again, with disastrous consequences. The total effect results in myocardial infarction—heart attack.

Heart Attack Prevention

Fortunately, now that we are beginning to understand the true cause of most heart attacks, we are better equipped to prevent them. Preventive strategies such as lowering the LDL (bad) cholesterol, strengthening the arterial walls, preventing platelets from clotting and removing saturated fat from your diet can go a long way toward lowering your risk of a heart attack.

God has made provision for our health—even for the prevention of heart attacks—and one of the keys to this provision, which I have mentioned, can be found in His Word. Consider its significance to the health of your heart:

> *You must never eat any fat or blood.*
> —LEVITICUS 3:17, NLT

> *Then the LORD said to Moses, "Give the Israelites these instructions: You must never eat fat, whether from oxen or sheep or goats. The fat of an animal found dead or killed by a wild animal may never be eaten, though it may be used for any other purpose. Anyone who eats fat from an offering given to the LORD by fire must be cut off from the community. Even in your homes you must never eat the blood of any bird or animal. Anyone who eats blood must be cut off from the community."*
> —LEVITICUS 7:22–27, NLT

The life of any creature is in its blood.
—LEVITICUS 17:11, NLT

Have you ever noticed that many people have heart attacks shortly after they have finished consuming a huge meal, which is often full of fatty foods? There is a much higher rate of heart attacks in people who have just consumed a meal that is high in saturated (animal) fats or transfatty acids from hydrogenated or partially hydrogenated oils. This fact is especially true among people who already have underlying coronary disease.[3]

The reason for this is that the fats contained in the food cause the coronary arteries to constrict and shut off the flow of blood in an already narrowed artery. Lack of blood flow to the heart then causes a myocardial infarction, otherwise known as a heart attack.

I find it interesting that God gave us instructions to keep us healthy in His written Word, which was written thousands of years ago. His command that we should never eat the fat or blood from an animal is now understood scientifically as a helpful prohibition to avoid the saturated fats found in meat—the fats known to be the most harmful to human beings. Other fats that God does not prohibit—fats found in certain vegetable oils, for example—have been found to be good for human consumption. The cultures that eat primarily these foods are remarkably healthier than those that consume primarily animal fat. Again, modern science proves that God knows what He is doing!

In His mercy, God continues to provide natural ways of healing for those who violate His command regarding the consumption of animal fat. There are two substances that, when taken with a fatty meal, will help prevent the constriction of arteries: vitamin E and oatmeal. Eight hundred international units of vitamin E (D-alpha variety) can help stop the artery constriction that usually takes place after the consumption of a fatty meal. I generally recommend the vitamin E supplement because it is so much easier to take than eating a bowl of oatmeal after a steak dinner. I also recommend reducing your intake of these harmful fats, if not eliminating them altogether.

Congestive heart failure

Congestive heart failure occurs when there has been so much damage to the heart muscle that it cannot pump fast enough to prevent a buildup of fluid in the lungs. Many people with congestive heart failure also have swelling or edema in their ankles. These patients usually reach a point where their lung capacity is so limited that they cannot lie flat in bed because when they do, it is difficult to breathe. They also become out of breath quickly with any level of exertion.

Long before doctors understood what congestive heart failure was, they knew that a certain family of plants—the rose family, which includes *hawthorn extract*—was helpful in strengthening the contractions of the heart. Today, we are rediscovering the uses of this invaluable natural substance.

Controlled studies have been conducted that show the benefits of hawthorn extract in the reversal of congestive heart failure. It has a direct effect on the electrical impulses of the heart, shortening the refractory time between heartbeats and allowing the heart to pump more fluid more effectively.[4]

Prevention of Heart Disease

The best way to stop heart attacks from occurring is to prevent heart disease from developing altogether. There are many new breakthrough discoveries from the natural plant kingdom that are causing great strides in the prevention of cardiovascular disease. Perhaps the most astounding of these is *policosanol.*

Policosanol

For years, people have been harvesting sugarcane in order to create that sweet substance so many of us use inordinately and that is actually very harmful to our bodies. In the production of sugar from sugarcane, an amazing by-product is created that until recently was considered simply a waste product. It is called *policosanol,* a waxy substance now determined to be a potent cholesterol-lowering and heart-protective agent. One study showed that it lowered the LDL (bad) cholesterol levels in patients 20 percent in just six to twelve weeks, rivaling the prescription medications Zocor, Lipitor and Pravachol—and *without the side effects of the prescription medications!*[5]

Many of these cholesterol medications cause the sudden onset of muscle aches and pains, which can progress into a breakdown of muscle tissue. They can also cause serious liver damage. Policosanol caused none of these side effects. (The only side effect noted was weight loss—and none of the subjects complained about that!) In addition, policosanol was shown to raise the levels of HDL (good) cholesterol by 15 percent. The recommended daily dose for policosanol is 10 milligrams.

God so often chooses the foolish things of the world to confound the wise. Who would have thought that a waste product of sugarcane could have such unbelievable healing properties? When you compare the side effects and the cost of prescription drugs to the good results possible with a natural substance like policosanol, it becomes clear that God is providing the healing for His people that He promised in His Word.

Natural treatments for homocysteine

One major new risk factor in the development of heart disease is the presence of homocysteine levels in the blood because they are so strongly associated with arterial blockage. In fact, many doctors consider high levels of homocysteine as great a risk factor for heart disease as smoking. However, once again, God has provided some natural remedies that help to lower the homocysteine levels in the blood.

Anyone with high homocysteine levels should be on a regimen of B_6 and B_{12} vitamins, as well as folic acid. Additionally, the chemical compound *trimethylglycine,* also known as *betaine,* has been shown to work in conjunction with the B vitamins in lowering homocysteine levels. Betaine actually is a methyl donor that is found in sugar beets.

Take 10 milligrams of vitamin B_6, 100 micrograms of vitamin B_{12} and 250 milligrams of betaine per day.

L-arginine

L-arginine, which helps to stimulate the production of nitric oxide in the body, should be included in any supplement program to protect the arteries. Nitric oxide is a natural chemical that dilates, or expands, the blood vessels in the body, including the coronary arteries. It is a good way to help increase the blood flow in blocked arteries or prevent blockage by keeping them expanded. L-arginine is also good to take after a fatty meal. As I stated previously, saturated fats cause the constriction of blood vessels, but taking L-arginine can counteract this effect. L-arginine should be taken at a dose of 1,000 milligrams per day.

Tocotrienols

Tocotrienols are actually cousins of vitamin E; they can be found in rice and rice bran. When taken in conjunction with policosanol, tocotrienols work even better than vitamin E to lower cholesterol and prevent platelets from sticking to the walls of the arteries. A mixed tocotrienol complex should be taken at a dose of 100 milligrams per day.

Garlic

Garlic is an effective cholesterol-lowering agent when used in combination with the other substances we have listed. Garlic bulb extract should be taken at a dose of 120 milligrams per day.

Green tea

Drinking one cup of green tea per day has an effect on blood vessel walls, making them more elastic and better able to expand to allow a free flow of blood. Obviously, this can significantly lower a person's risk of developing heart disease or suffering a stroke.

 ASK DR. CHERRY

QUESTION: **Sometimes when I lie in bed at night, I can hear my heart beating very loudly, like a constant pulsing in my head. Is there something wrong with me?**

ANSWER: Many people who lie on their sides or stomach to sleep at night experience a pounding heartbeat, and they begin to worry that they are about to have a stroke or that something dire is wrong with them. In fact, this is a completely normal phenomenon. There is a small artery that runs by the inner ear, off of the carotid artery, and if you are lying in just the right position and there are no other noises around you, you can hear the blood pulsing quite loudly through that branch in the artery.

QUESTION: **What is the best way to take my pulse?**

ANSWER: Sometimes if the pulse in a person's wrist is weak, medical personnel will take the pulse in the neck. However, I would not recommend that you do so for one important reason. If you have a slight stenosis, or narrowing, of your carotid artery, and if there is a small calcium deposit present there, by pushing around in that area to find a pulse, you may inadvertently dislodge the calcium deposit and send it through your bloodstream straight to your brain. I always encourage my patients to take their pulse at the wrist. It may take a little practice, but you can do it. Begin to take it often, when you are resting comfortably and seated, to determine what your usual resting heart rate is.

QUESTION: **If I already experience irregular heartbeats, should I increase the dosages of natural supplements that you recommended in order to take control of the disease?**

ANSWER: This is a good question, and the answer depends on the frequency of the problem. Most people who are concerned with just preventing problems can get by with the dosages I recommended, but a person who is experiencing severe difficulties may need to double or even triple the coenzyme Q_{10}, for example. Be sure to check with your own doctor so that your treatment and condition can be monitored as you use these supplements.

ESSENTIAL NUTRIENTS FOR A HEALTHY HEART

NUTRIENT	EFFECT	DAILY DOSAGE
L-arginine	Amino acid important in blood vessel regulation and cardiac function	1,000 mg
Betaine	Nutrient that protects the heart by regulating homocysteine levels	250 mg
Coenzyme Q_{10}	Nutrient essential to energy production in the heart and muscles	50 mg
Garlic bulb extract	Herb with numerous phyto-chemicals that help normalize blood pressure, reduce platelet stickiness and regulate blood lipid levels	120 mg
Green tea leaf extract	Natural source of catechin antioxidants that protect tissues from free-radical damage	150 mg
Magnesium	Mineral concentrated in heart tissue and needed for energy metabolism in the heart	400 mg
Policosanol	Plant derivative that supports healthy cholesterol levels	10 mg

NUTRIENT	EFFECT	DAILY DOSAGE
Mixed tocotrienol complex	Part of the vitamin E complex with important antioxidant and cholesterol-regulating activity	100 mg
Vitamin B$_6$	Essential vitamin that protects the heart by lowering homocysteine levels	10 mg
Vitamin B$_{12}$	Essential vitamin that protects the heart by lowering homocysteine levels	100 mcg
Potassium	Helps regulate heart rhythms	99 mg
Calcium	Stabilizes heart rates and lowers blood pressure	500 mg

CHAPTER 6

LOWER BLOOD
PRESSURE–NATURALLY

*He will redeem their life from oppression and vio-
lence; and precious shall be their blood in His sight.*
—PSALM 72:14, NKJV

HIGH BLOOD PRESSURE IS ACCURATELY CALLED THE *SILENT KILLER.* It is
often the root cause of many other health problems, especially heart
disease. As blood pressure readings approach 140/90 and above, a silent
but deadly process begins weakening the body. Strain is placed on the heart
muscle, and thickening in the pumping chamber of the heart (left ventricular hypertrophy) occurs. The incidence of heart attack and stroke begins
to increase, and the kidneys begin suffering damage.

Many people believe that if their blood pressure is up, they will have
some visible sign such as headaches or nosebleeds—but these are the
exception. Usually there is no warning of high blood pressure until something breaks. By then it is a major battle to overcome the problem.

Unfortunately, even when high blood pressure—also known as *hypertension*—is caught in time, many of the medications used by medical doctors
to lower it have detrimental side effects, are rather expensive even with
health insurance and can be dangerous when combined with other drugs
or certain foods.

God has a better way! The Bible tells us that "the leaves of the tree were for the healing of the nations" (Rev. 22:2, NKJV). There are three natural supplements that, when used on a daily basis, can lower blood pressure naturally *and with no side effects!*

Potassium

There are many studies that indicate the power of potassium to reduce blood pressure. I have found potassium to effectively protect the kidneys also because of its role in protecting the lining of blood vessels from damage. Consuming five or more servings of fruits and vegetables daily is the ideal way to obtain sufficient potassium. We also recommend potassium in the citrate form at a total of 99 milligrams daily. Taking the supplement will ensure constant blood levels, and your dietary intake of fruits and vegetables can simply build on this consistent level.

Polyphenols

Polyphenols are important compounds found in numerous foods. One particular association has been reported between certain polyphenols found in olive oil and the lowering of blood pressure.

A study reported in one medical journal noted that patients using 1–2 tablespoons of olive oil daily showed a marked reduction in the required dosage of blood pressure medications.[1] In fact, patients who were on antihypertensive medications were frequently able to cut their medicine dosage in half after only a few months.

In these studies, a cold-pressed, extra-virgin olive oil was utilized. Other oils, such as polyunsaturated oils, do not have these polyphenols present and do not produce a reduction in blood pressure. The compounds contained in the olive oil stimulate the production of a natural substance, known as *nitric oxide,* already present in the human body.

Nitric oxide is important because it tends to relax and dilate blood vessels, which results in blood pressure reduction. These phenols also function as antioxidants that reduce the damaging effects of free-radical compounds that can affect blood vessels.

Amazingly, almost one-fourth of the patients in this study who were using olive oil were able to control their blood pressure without any prescription drugs![2] It is interesting to note that olive oil is an important component of the Mediterranean diet. This may be one of many reasons that countries around the Mediterranean region have some of the lowest recorded rates of heart disease in the world.

Magnesium

Magnesium is an increasingly important mineral. Recent studies conducted at Harvard University that looked at health habits among health professionals found that those who consumed higher amounts of magnesium in the form of fruits and vegetables had significantly lower blood pressure.[3]

Another study, known as the Honolulu Heart Study, showed that magnesium was the most consistent substance that correlated with lowering the systolic and diastolic (upper and lower) blood pressure. (Systolic blood pressure is the pressure that occurs when the heart beats; diastolic blood pressure measures the relaxation of the heart between beats.) This study consistently showed that the lower the blood magnesium levels, the higher the risk of heart attacks and the development of high blood pressure.[4]

Low magnesium levels also correlated with hardening of the arteries and the accumulation of cholesterol plaque in the carotid arteries, which supply blood to the brain. Increased magnesium intake causes blood vessels to dilate, which, in turn, results in reduced blood pressure.

Over the past several decades, the dietary intake of magnesium in the United States has decreased by slightly over 50 percent. At the same time, we are facing an epidemic of high blood pressure, with approximately 55 million Americans currently diagnosed with hypertension.[5]

Because of this epidemic, the time has come for magnesium supplementation. In fact, studies have been done using magnesium as a daily supplement. These studies indicated that both the systolic and diastolic blood pressures fell significantly during the period of the supplemental intake.[6]

Magnesium can also help prevent heart palpitations and improve cholesterol levels. Even greater benefits are noted when the magnesium is taken with a potassium supplement and when salt is restricted in the diet.

Yes, We Have No Bananas!

It is incredible to think that such a popular fruit as the banana can actually function as a blood-pressure-lowering agent, but more and more studies are pointing in that direction. We have known for some time that potassium can lower blood pressure to some extent and that bananas are high in potassium. More startling, however, is the recent discovery that bananas contain a natural compound used in our most popular antihypertensive medications!

One of the most popular classes of antihypertensives (blood pressure medications) is known as ACE inhibitors or ACE blockers. These are prescribed by physicians and rank near the top of the list for treating patients with high blood pressure, patients who have had heart attacks and patients with congestive heart failure.

This class of drugs has also shown a protective effect on the kidneys of patients suffering kidney problems from diabetes. In fact, this is one of the safest types of blood pressure medication you can take. It is available in a one-pill-a-day dose form, and the newer varieties of the ACE blockers have almost no side effects.

The latest studies indicate that bananas contain a natural ACE blocker and can lower blood pressure up to 10 percent in patients who consume two bananas daily.[7]

Take Action!

Because high blood pressure can creep up slowly on a person, giving no warning signs until it is too late, it is so important to be proactive in preventing potential serious problems before they strike. *Have your blood pressure checked regularly.* If your doctor sees readings in the 130/80 range, it is time to take action. You should lose weight, exercise, increase your consumption of fruit—especially bananas—and consider taking supplements that can lower blood pressure, including garlic capsules (the equivalent of one clove daily).

If your readings are found to be consistently over 140/90, you may need to be on a one-pill-a-day prescription drug such as one of the ACE drugs. Once you start taking a drug, this does not mean that you will be on it for life. When lifestyle changes are made, many patients can decrease and even go off their blood pressure medicine. However, this must be done with close monitoring under the care of a physician.

ASK DR. CHERRY

QUESTION: **Is grapefruit juice OK to drink while I am taking blood pressure medications?**

ANSWER: No. Most people do not realize that a chemical in grapefruit juice will increase the blood levels of many medications. This is especially dangerous with blood pressure medications as they need to be monitored so closely. If you are taking blood pressure or any other medication, ask your doctor about the interactive effects of grapefruit juice with those drugs. There are many benefits of grapefruit juice, but they can be achieved in other ways through the use of supplements if the juice itself would be harmful to you.

QUESTION: **If I am taking a prescription blood thinner to prevent a possible stroke, what supplements am I allowed to take? I have heard that some of them also have a blood-thinning effect.**

ANSWER: Certain supplements, such as vitamin E, St. John's wort and ginkgo biloba, have blood-thinning properties in them. If you are already taking a prescription blood thinner, such as Coumadin, you should start these supplements slowly and carefully, and be sure to have your blood checked frequently so that you do not develop a tendency to bleed. However, many of my patients who begin to take these supplements find that they are able to eventually decrease their prescription medication. Any such changes should, however, take place under your own doctor's care and supervision.

CHAPTER 7

PREVENT HARDENING OF THE ARTERIES

Heal me, O LORD, and I shall be healed; save me,
and I shall be saved, for You are my praise.
—JEREMIAH 17:14, NKJV

NEXT TO *CANCER,* HARDENING OF THE ARTERIES IS ONE OF OUR MOST SERIOUS CONCERNS. This disease, also known as *atherosclerosis,* is, in fact, the leading cause of heart attacks and strokes, which kill more people in industrialized countries than all forms of cancer combined.[1] Is there anything we can do to stop this process, or is it just "in our genes," an inevitable part of aging? There are multiple things you can do to avoid facing this ravaging problem.

Scientists are finding that hardening of the arteries is really an inflammation in the arteries. Most of us think that hardening of the arteries is a condition in which solid calcium deposits form in the arteries just as calcium forms in the water pipes in our homes. This is not an accurate understanding of what is occurring.

The LDL (bad) cholesterol forms a solid or semi-solid plaque or deposit that can stiffen artery walls. This plaque consists of white blood cells, smooth muscle cells, platelets and other components, but it basically represents an inflammatory process in the plaque. There are at least four approaches you can take to help prevent this deadly problem from attacking your body.

Take Low-Dose Aspirin

Amazingly, half of the people with these plaques, which can clog the arteries, have normal cholesterol levels. It is the initial damage to the artery lining caused by the bad cholesterol that sets the stage for inflammation. This is why one low-dose (81 milligrams) "enteric-coated" baby aspirin can work wonders in preventing heart disease—it stops the inflammation. (The term "enteric-coated" should appear on the label of the bottle.) Interestingly, regular aspirin (325 milligrams) may not be as effective as the low-dose aspirin (81 milligrams).

Take Antioxidants

Why does the cholesterol damage the arteries? Damage is caused by the oxidation or breakdown of the LDL cholesterol, which enables it to harm the healthy cells lining the arteries. This is why it is so critical to provide antioxidants in the form of vitamin E (800 international units daily), vitamin C (2,000 milligrams daily), selenium (200 micrograms daily) along with others, such as the carotenes and coenzyme Q_{10}.

Lower Homocysteine Levels

Protein is another potential culprit in the development of atherosclerosis. It is not the protein we eat (which is good for us), but the breakdown of certain types of protein (amino acids) into a by-product known as *homocysteine* that can cause problems. High homocysteine levels can damage the arteries, and these levels increase when we lack sufficient amounts of B vitamins in our diet.

To prevent hardening of the arteries, I recommend that you take 600 micrograms of folic acid daily, 75 milligrams of vitamin B_6 daily and 100 micrograms of vitamin B_{12} daily. These amounts of B vitamins keep the homocysteine levels low and thus offer sufficient protection from hardening of the arteries.

Policicosanol

Policosanol is a chemical derived from sugarcane that has been found effective in reducing cholesterol levels. To prevent atherosclerosis, the LDL (bad) levels of cholesterol need to be under 100, and the HDL (good) levels of cholesterol should be well above 40.

Please don't take the attitude that hardening of the arteries could never happen to you. The Scriptures declare that "he who does not use his endeavors to heal himself is brother to him who commits suicide" (Prov. 18:9, AMP). Do what you can to prevent atherosclerosis *before* it happens so that you can live a long and fruitful life.

ASK DR. CHERRY

QUESTION: **Are there any side effects to the use of policicosanol?**

ANSWER: Most prescription medications that are prescribed to prevent the hardening of the arteries have numerous adverse side effects, but the substances that are gleaned from God's plant kingdom generally have none. Policosanol is a substance that is actually gleaned from the root of the sugarcane, and its only known side effect is that it causes many patients to lose weight—something that most people don't complain about!

QUESTION: **How great of a risk factor for atherosclerosis is the presence of homocysteine in the blood?**

ANSWER: One major risk factor in the development of atherosclerosis, and therefore in the progression of heart disease and the possibility of a stroke, is the presence of homocysteine levels in the blood. In fact, many doctors now consider high levels of homocysteine as great a risk factor as smoking for heart disease. It is so important to do whatever possible to keep your homocysteine levels low.

CHAPTER 8

BALANCING THE IMMUNE SYSTEM

*Surely He shall deliver you from the snare of
the fowler and from the perilous pestilence...
No evil shall befall you, nor shall any
plague come near your dwelling.*
—PSALM 91:3, 10, NKJV

GOD PROMISES TO PROTECT HIS PEOPLE. Psalm 91 contains a beautiful description of the blessings of protection that God has made available to His children. Not only does God's protection shield us from our spiritual enemies, but also part of His blessing is protection from any *plagues* or *pestilence* that might try to come upon us. Plagues and pestilence signify disease, but God's children don't have to fear such contagion, for we are promised a satisfying, lengthy life. Take a moment to read the comforting promises God gives to us in several verses of this psalm:

*He who dwells in the secret place of the Most High shall abide
under the shadow of the Almighty. I will say of the LORD, "He is
my refuge and my fortress; my God, in Him I will trust." Surely
He shall deliver you from the snare of the fowler and from the
perilous pestilence...Because you have made the LORD, who is
my refuge, even the Most High, your dwelling place, no evil shall
befall you, nor shall any plague come near your dwelling; for He
shall give His angels charge over you, to keep you in all your*

63

ways…"Because he has set his love upon Me, therefore I will deliver him; I will set him on high, because he has known My name. He shall call upon Me, and I will answer him; I will be with him in trouble; I will deliver him and honor him. With long life I will satisfy him, and show him My salvation."
PSALM 91:1–3, 9–11, 14–16, NKJV

Protection From Plagues and Pestilence

One way God chooses to protect us from disease is through the natural immune system that He built into our bodies. It is our "hedge of protection" between our bodies and the harmful bacteria and viruses that are present in the world. Because the Christian's body is, quite literally, the temple of the Holy Spirit (1 Cor. 6:19), how much more should we protect it from harm? By learning how our bodies function, as well as how to keep our immune systems balanced and working properly, we will be able to fight off the many diseases that are rampant in our world today and thus receive God's promise of a long and healthy life.

Unfortunately, many people suffer from one or more diseases, the causes of which they really don't understand. The list of illnesses that spring from an imbalance in the immune system runs a virtual gamut of "plagues," including asthma, rheumatoid arthritis, moderate to severe allergies, inflammatory bowel disease (including Crohn's disease), Hodgkin's disease, leukemia and even more dreaded forms of cancer.

How can you begin to implement God's promises of protection against plagues and pestilence into the daily world in which you live? You must begin to follow His commands for healthy eating patterns that will bring your immune system back into the balance He created it to have.

Diseases of the Immune System

Diseases of the immune system fall into three primary categories:

- Illnesses that result from an overactive immune system

- Illnesses that result from an underactive immune system

- Diseases that indicate the immune system has turned on the body and is attacking itself

To gain an understanding of what happens when things go awry in your immune system, first take a look at how it was designed to function.

The human body contains a vast array of various kinds of cells—white blood cells, lymphocytes, T-cells and natural killer cells—all designed to ward off any invasions of the body, especially those that would cause a catastrophic illness. Scientists call certain kinds of cells "natural killer cells" because their job is to hunt down and kill these foreign invaders that cause disease. One of these types of killer cells is called a *macrophage*, meaning "big eater." God created this cell to devour, much like Pac-Man in the old video arcade game, any dangerous or foreign substances that enter the body.

Proper functioning of the T-cells is very important because they act as the "commanders of the army," directing the macrophages into battle. God's promise in Psalm 91 is realized through the macrophages already present in your own body. Every time you successfully fight off a cold, for example, you can thank God for His Word and that His promises are always true—your immune system has turned away yet another plague from your dwelling place—and His!

So many times, when people think of diseases of the immune system, they jump to the conclusion that these diseases occur when the immune system has somehow been compromised or knocked out altogether. A classic example of this would be the AIDS virus, which results in the immune system becoming deficient and underactive, leaving the person vulnerable to any number of contagious and deadly diseases. AIDS itself is not what kills a person; the diseases to which the person is helplessly exposed strike the fatal blow because of an underactive immune system.

An underactive immune system is not the only way the body becomes compromised. If the body's immune system becomes *overactive,* serious problems can also occur, and if it reaches the point where the body's defenses begin to *attack itself,* a whole new category of illnesses, referred to as *autoimmune disorders,* is the result. A closer look at these three problems will help you know how to walk toward healing.

Underactive immune system

When the immune system is no longer capable of stopping an attack, the person becomes vulnerable to all types of terrible "plagues." If you are someone who frequently catches colds or has difficulty getting over them, your immune system could be compromised in some way. Respiratory infections, viral infections—including the West Nile virus that caused such a stir recently—and, of course, the ultimate failure of the immune system—cancer—belong in this first category of illnesses.

Did you know that every one of us develops a form of cancer once or twice a week throughout our entire lives? A "cancerous" cell is simply a cell that has gone astray—it begins to divide abnormally on its own until it has divided enough times to get out of control. Our immune systems are designed to recognize those cells as soon as an abnormal division takes place. Then our T-cells lead our macrophages ("big eaters") into battle to kill and eat up the cancer before it progresses. The cancers that go on to cause problems and eventually kill people are indicative of a failure of the immune system to catch the problem in time.

Overactive immune system

Many people believe that the more active their immune system is, the better off they are, but that is not the case. Sometimes the body becomes so "paranoid" about potential invasion that it begins to recognize harmless substances as foreign invaders to be attacked, sometimes with great fervor. Moderate or severe allergies are classic examples of this phenomenon. When something harmless, such as a miniscule dust mite or piece of pollen, is breathed in, the immune system, sensing grave danger, begins to send a flood of histamine on the attack to squeeze liquid out of the cells and flush the foreign particle out of the system. This is what causes the sneezing, wheezing, coughing and runny eyes and nose that make people miserable.

Other diseases that demonstrate this overactivity include asthma—in which the body's reaction is wheezing and shortness of breath—and chronic fatigue syndrome or fibromyalgia—in which the body responds with fatigue and a total lack of energy.

Autoimmune disorders

Sometimes the body's immune system goes totally "haywire," and, instead of attacking a foreign invader, it begins to attack the body itself. In multiple sclerosis, for example, the body literally attacks the myelin sheath that lines the nerve endings. In inflammatory bowel disease, including Crohn's disease and ileitis, the body attacks its own lower digestive tract. Other diseases in this category include lupus, rheumatoid arthritis and scleroderma.

Interestingly, autoimmune diseases are much more common among women than they are among men, possibly due to a hormonal relationship of which we are not yet fully aware.

We've Missed the Root Cause

Traditional medicine typically attempts to treat these diseases individually by coming up with a new antibiotic to combat viruses, new nasal sprays to alleviate allergy symptoms or new treatments to shrink cancerous tumors. While these treatments have their place, none of them are dealing with the root cause: an immune system that is out of balance.

How many times have you been treated for a recurring virus with another round of antibiotics? That has become such a pat answer for most infections that it doesn't even occur to some doctors that it might not be the best solution. Antibiotics can be harmful to our bodies because they not only kill the "bad" bacteria but also the "good" bacteria, or flora, in our intestines that help promote healthy immune system function.

The times in which we live today are dangerous ones, as the threat of bioterrorism has become increasingly real in the last several years. The fear used to be that some diseases such as smallpox might accidentally reappear, but now the fear is that they will be released on the world intentionally. In addition, new strains of viruses that have never before been reported in the United States are now on the rise, such as the West Nile virus and the Ebola virus, two of the most deadly.

In the development of "cures" for these diseases, traditional medicine inadvertently can create as much harm as good: For years the drug methicillin was used to kill off the deadly *Staphylococcus* bacteria, but now much of these bacteria have become resistant to the drug. What are we to do? How can we protect ourselves? It is not time to become hopeless or to lose heart. It is time to remember the promises of Psalm 91—God has not left us defenseless.

In these last days, God is beginning to bring awareness to the medical community of the root cause of many of the diseases that plague millions of Americans. Giving proper attention to the immune system can bring the answer to health we are searching for. The answer does not necessarily lie in stimulating, or "revving up," the immune systems of patients across the board. Although there are cases in which its ability to recognize and wipe out disease needs to be increased, other cases require a *decrease* in immune system function. When people take certain products inappropriately to enhance their immunity or overuse antibiotics to try to prevent infections, they run the risk of developing other serious problems, such as asthma and allergies or, even worse, some of the devastating autoimmune disorders.

Putting "Glasses" on the Immune System

The key, as it is with many things in God's kingdom, is *balance*. Our goal must be to restore our immune system to a healthy balance, in which it responds correctly to dangerous situations but lets harmless particles through without a fuss.

I like to describe the restoration of this balance as *putting glasses on the immune system*. For example, if you have poor vision, you are unable to recognize things clearly. When someone knocks on your door, you may squint through the peephole, see someone who looks like your best friend, and then swing open the door—only to welcome an intruder. Or if you see someone on the street who looks like an enemy, you may try to defend yourself, not realizing that it is a friend you're attacking.

Perhaps that seems like an extreme example, but that is what the immune system is doing in many of these diseases. Like a person suffering with poor vision, it has lost the ability to distinguish between friend and foe. So what we want to do is put glasses on the immune system—restore its vision, its ability to recognize true danger, and respond appropriately. The key to that process is balance.

Nutrients That Protect and Restore Proper Immune System Function

A natural decline in immune system function takes place in every person as they age, beginning as early as the thirties, due to a deficiency in certain nutrients throughout life. That is why every person, regardless of whether or not they are demonstrating symptoms of any of these diseases, should be protecting their immune systems with nutritional supplements. I have listed below the common nutrient along with proper dosages to take to ensure a healthy immune system throughout your life span.

Vitamin E
I recommend 800 international units daily to protect the immune system.

Tocotrienols
The tocotrienols are "cousins" of vitamin E and are essential for vitamin E to work properly. I recommend 105 milligrams of tocotrienols daily.

Vitamin C
Vitamin C is critical for lymphocyte function, which is why it is good to drink orange juice when you have a cold. I recommend 2 grams of vitamin C (2,000 milligrams) per day.

Zinc

To simply protect the immune system, I recommend 15 milligrams per day. Use caution, however, when taking zinc, as it affects the absorption of copper in the body. It would be best to take zinc in the form of a multi-vitamin that also supplements copper, for if you increase your zinc intake without also increasing copper, you may become copper-deficient. And because copper is necessary for white blood cell function, any deficiencies will adversely affect the immune system—the very opposite of the effect you originally intended to achieve!

Additionally, too much zinc in the system will interfere with immune system function, so be sure to avoid the misconception that "more is better." That is not always the case! Please take only the dosages that are recommended, and you will avoid a host of unnecessary problems.

Beta carotene

Beta carotene is transformed by the body into vitamin A, known to strengthen the immune system. Beta carotene is preferable to taking higher doses of vitamin A, which can affect liver function. The body will take the beta carotene it receives and only manufacture the vitamin A that it needs from that. I recommend 20,000 international units a day.

Selenium

Selenium is a mineral that has been shown to be critical to the immune system by stimulating our "natural killer" cells that attack harmful viruses or cancers. It also balances the immune system to work more effectively. One study done over a period of ten years looked at the immune systems of thirteen hundred people who took 200 micrograms of selenium a day. The rates of cancer development (every type of cancer) in this group of people dropped 40 percent, and the rates of lung, prostate and colon cancer specifically were reduced by 50 percent![1] For this reason, I recommend 200 micrograms daily.

Author's note

If you are facing one of the diseases we listed that is related to a malfunctioning immune system, it is necessary to increase the dosages of the nutrients listed below to the given levels:

~ *Vitamin E:* Increase to 1,000 international units daily.

~ *Tocotrienols:* Continue taking 105 milligrams per day.

~ *Vitamin C:* Increase to 2,500 milligrams per day.

∽ *Zinc:* Increase (cautiously) to 25 milligrams per day. Be sure to increase your copper intake as well to maintain a healthy balance.

∽ *Beta carotene:* Increase to 25,000 international units per day.

∽ *Selenium:* Increase to 320 micrograms per day.

Herbal Preparations to Enhance the Immune System

Numerous herbs have been found within God's plant kingdom that restore balance to the immune system. Most modern prescriptions that man has devised for immune system function *either* slow down *or* stimulate the immune system; they do not work to balance it. God's natural substances do both, slowing and stimulating as needed; His purpose is balance in all things. The natural herbs listed below are God's provision for enhancing the immune system.

Pomegranate seed

Pomegranates have been around at least since biblical times. Studies from Israel are now reporting that pomegranate extract triggers a self-destruction mechanism in breast cancer cells. It is the first time that a common ingredient has been found to stimulate the immune system to attack cancer in the body.[2] My recommendation is 50 milligrams per day.

Elderberry

Another study from researchers in Israel examined the effect of elderberry on common viral influenzas. Elderberry performed two functions: It directly inhibited the virus itself, and it stimulated the immune system to attack the virus more vigorously. The effect was that flu symptoms were reduced by 50 percent.[3] I recommend common elderberry in the extract form, 100 milligrams a day.

Astragalus

Astragalus promotes an increase in the number of T-cells ("commanders of the army") in the body, boosting resistance to infection and, even more importantly, countering the age-related decline that all of us see in our immune systems. As we get older, our T-cell counts decline, most commonly due to poor dietary habits and the polluted environment, but astragalus overcomes that decline and can restore the immune system to that of a twenty-year-old. I recommend 100 milligrams a day.

Beta 1,3 glucans

Beta 1,3 glucans are polysaccharide compounds, a type of complex carbohydrate commonly found in the cell walls of baker's yeast and also found in a slightly different form in mushrooms. Like some of the other substances I have mentioned, beta glucans stimulate a weakened immune system, but will not overstimulate it (unlike many prescription medications that do). Beta glucans strengthen the macrophage ("big eaters") function and have been shown to significantly reduce the risk of postoperative infections. The daily recommended dose is 25 milligrams per day.

Mushrooms

Mushrooms promote healthy immune systems because they contain beta 1,3 glucans. There are three main classifications of mushrooms, each of which originated in Asia, all having slightly different healing properties. The *maitake* mushroom has been called the "king of the mushrooms." According to one study performed in China, the maitake mushroom both inhibited cancerous tumors from forming and killed cancer cells associated with lung, stomach and liver cancer by stimulating the T-cells and the macrophages.[4] The *reishi* mushroom has been shown effective in the treatment of allergies and asthma by bringing an overstimulated immune system back into balance and inhibiting the release of histamine against harmless agents. The *shiitake* mushroom contains an unusual compound called lentinon, which is extremely potent in balancing the immune system and in the prevention of cancer. It is so potent, in fact, that it is currently being studied as a potential treatment for the HIV/AIDS virus.

Garlic

Garlic is used for many different reasons as it affects multiple body systems. It has been found to alter cholesterol levels and enhance the cardiovascular system in addition to its benefits to the immune system. There are thirty different cancer-fighting compounds in garlic alone.

If you are wondering about how to implement all of these nutrients into your diet in a tasty way, please try the recipe for "Cancer-Fighting Lentil Soup" that my wife, Linda, has developed; it is delicious. (See Appendix B.) In addition to making changes in your diet to consume natural nutrients, I also recommend that you supply your body with the supplements we have discussed that will restore balance to your immune system.

The Synergistic Effect

You will see the greatest effect in the restoration of your immune system when you combine these supplemental nutrients and common herbs and incorporate them into a more natural, healthy diet. They will work together in your body to balance your immune system so that it can provide resistance against viruses, harmful bacteria and cancer, as well as preventing it from attacking harmless substances or even your own body.

If you have any of the diseases that have been discussed in this chapter, let me encourage you to begin a three-pronged attack against them:

> *Pray* that God would put "glasses" on your immune system so that it will recognize and attack only the things it was intended to attack.

> *Read the Word.* Begin to speak Psalm 91 over your life, declaring the promises for protection from plagues and pestilence and for a long and satisfying life.

> *Supplement.* Begin a regimen of supplementing your healthy diet with these nutrients and herbs and with other protocol from advice you receive in this book for a healthy lifestyle.

ASK DR. CHERRY

QUESTION: **When should I take an antibiotic?**

ANSWER: Antibiotics should be taken sparingly. Of course, if a person is suffering from a serious bacterial infection such as pneumonia, antibiotics may be necessary to bring the illness under control. However, overly prescribing antibiotics can lead to some strains of bacteria becoming resistant to its effects. Also, because antibiotics kill both "good" and "bad" bacteria in the body, they will disrupt the healthy balance of necessary flora, especially in the intestines. After any round of antibiotics, a supplement such as lactobacillus should be taken to restore the "good" bacteria in the body.

QUESTION: **I have heard that green tea can be helpful for people who have cancer. Is this true?**

ANSWER: It's no coincidence that people in Asia, where green tea is a very popular drink, have one of the lowest incidences of cancer in the world. Green tea contains polyphenols, which do, in fact, prevent cancer from developing; if cancer occurs, they also fight against it.

Incidentally, the people of the world who have the lowest cancer rates are those cultures whose primary diet is the "Mediterranean diet." You may be aware that the Mediterranean diet generally follows the principles outlined in the Old Testament dietary laws. Because they do not violate God's principles for health, they have a great degree of protection against such a devastating disease as cancer.

ESSENTIAL NUTRIENTS FOR A BALANCED IMMUNE SYSTEM

NUTRIENT	EFFECT	DAILY DOSAGE	TREATMENT DOSAGE
Astragalus root powder	Herb widely used in traditional Chinese medicine to provide immune support	50 mg	100 mg
Beta glucan	Naturally derived plant substance known to boost immune function	25 mg	25 mg
Elderberry fruit powder	Herb traditionally used to support healthy respiratory and immune function	50 mg	100 mg
Garlic bulb extract	Herb widely used as a natural antimicrobial and immune enhancer	100 mg	100 mg
Maitake mushroom	Herb traditionally used as an aid to healthy immune and liver function	25 mg	25 mg
Pomegranate fruit extract	Herbal extract rich in antioxidant flavonoids	25 mg	50 mg
Reishi mushroom	Herb that contains a broad spectrum of antioxidant, detoxifying and immunomodulating substances	5 mg	5 mg
Selenium	Essential mineral that enhances many aspects of immune function and helps protect against a number of chronic diseases	200 mcg	320 mcg

ESSENTIAL NUTRIENTS FOR A BALANCED IMMUNE SYSTEM

NUTRIENT	EFFECT	DAILY DOSAGE	TREATMENT DOSAGE
Shiitake mushroom	Herb rich in immunomodulating substances that has been widely used in China and Japan for its immune-enhancing effects	5 mg	5 mg
Mixed tocotrienol complex	Important component of vitamin E with potent antioxidant activity	105 mg	105 mg
Beta carotene	Essential vitamin that plays an important role in maintaining a healthy immune system	20,000 IU	25,000 IU
Vitamin C	Essential vitamin that enhances the body's natural resistance to invasion by harmful microorganisms	2,000 mg	2,500 mg
Zinc	Essential mineral that boosts immune function and has been shown in studies to reduce the duration and severity of respiratory infections	15 mg	25 mg
Vitamin E	Essential vitamin that protects the immune system	800 IU	1,000 IU

CHAPTER 9

PROTECT YOURSELF FROM COLDS & FLU

I will put none of the diseases on you which
I have brought on the Egyptians. For I am
the LORD who heals you.
—EXODUS 15:26, NKJV

EVERYBODY HAS HAD IT AT LEAST A FEW TIMES. And when you see the clerk at the grocery store sneezing and coughing as she scans your merchandise, you realize that it could be coming your way soon.

Perhaps the most common ailments in the world are colds and flu viruses. We generally consider them just a nuisance to be endured, especially at certain times of the year. But if there were a way to prevent this misery and avoid the irritation and the loss of days of being productive in God's kingdom, wouldn't it be worth pursuing? For years, scientists have been working on the elusive "cure" for the common cold, which they have yet to discover. Fortunately, there are several natural ways to *prevent* it and to help protect yourself from ever catching a cold or coming down with the flu in the first place.

Cold or Flu?

Because different viruses are involved in colds and the flu, it is helpful to recognize symptomatically which you are suffering. The following chart lists some of the common symptoms of each condition along with their intensity to help you differentiate between these common conditions.

SYMPTOMS	COLDS	FLU
Fever	Rare	Typical; high (102°–104° F); lasts three to four days
Headache	Rare	Prominent
General aches and pains	Light	Usual; often severe
Fatigue, weakness	Mild	Can last up to two to three weeks
Extreme exhaustion	Never	Early and prominent
Stuffy nose	Common	Sometimes
Sneezing	Usual	Sometimes
Sore throat	Common	Sometimes
Chest discomfort	Mild to moderate	Common; can become severe

Echinacea

Echinacea is familiar to many people as a popular immune-boosting herb. It ranks near the top of the list when it comes to countering colds or the flu. This herb not only prevents viral infections, but it can also fight them if they try to attack the body. Many of the patients that I see in my practice take echinacea during the cold and flu season simply as a preventive measure. Studies have demonstrated that it can shorten the duration of the common cold and help prevent the flu from developing.

Echinacea works by stimulating the immune system, but it should not be taken on a daily basis for an extended period of time because tolerance can develop and cause it not to work as effectively. Echinacea should be used for four to eight weeks and then discontinued for at least two weeks. The recommended dosage is 2 to 3 teaspoons of the tincture daily, or you can take the standard-dose capsules and follow the directions on the label.

Garlic

Another important herb to use during the cold and flu season is garlic, which can fight viruses as well as bacteria. It is also effective for reducing the duration of colds and the flu. Again, garlic works by stimulating the immune system function. I recommend taking the capsule form daily, checking the label to be certain a capsule is the equivalent of one clove of fresh garlic.

Lesser-known herbs

There are several lesser-known herbs that are helpful for colds and the flu. For example, *thyme* has antiviral as well as antibacterial properties and can be made into a tea or taken as syrup. Another herb available at health food stores, known as *elder*, is a decongestant and an anti-inflammatory that has traditionally been taken in the form of a hot tea. *Lemon balm* is a helpful herb for easing headaches and the aching associated with flu symptoms.

Be certain also that you are on a good supplement program with a multi-vitamin and mineral supplement that includes B complex, zinc and vitamin E, as well as chromium and selenium. All of these nutrients support immune system function. Remember the old chicken soup recipe? If you come down with symptoms, it can help to clear out mucus.

The body often develops a fever during a bout with the flu. Fevers stimulate the body's immune system and help it overcome the virus and bacterial infection. Of course, a fever that is too high can be dangerous, as we know. Be sure to force fluids, particularly if you have developed a fever. It is very important to do all you can to strengthen your body's defenses against these viral infections.

If you do come down with the flu despite all of your best natural efforts, there are now prescription treatments available for it, if taken within the first two days of symptom onset. Tamiflu, 75 milligrams twice daily, prescribed by your doctor, can dramatically decrease the flu symptoms.

Natural Sinus Treatments

If you are always tired, if you constantly experience postnasal drainage or feel that you have a cold all of the time, you could be afflicted with *chronic sinusitis*. It is important to distinguish an acute episode of sinusitis (inflammation of the sinus cavities) from chronic, persistent sinusitis.

Acute sinus problems begin with head congestion, thick green/yellow nasal drainage, postnasal mucus drainage and extreme fatigue. These cold symptoms can last two or more weeks. *Chronic sinus* problems are identified by a low-grade infection, with periodic episodes of acute sinusitis. Patients often feel "sick all the time." They can have episodes of acute sinusitis, with the abovementioned symptoms, and three or more infections within six months, feeling good between episodes.

A third category of sinus problems involves *chronic inflammation* of the mucous membranes of the nose and sinus area but few, if any, infections. Doctors often mistakenly treat chronic sinusitis patients with antibiotics on a regular basis. This overuse of antibiotics can only lead to resistant "bugs," and eventually even the most powerful antibiotics will prove ineffective.

In patients who have persistent low-grade infection, with periodic flare-ups of acute sinus problems and a feeling of being sick most of the time, antibiotics can be a real mistake, as they promote more infection and do not offer a cure. Overuse of antibiotics can actually contribute to the inflammation that aggravates the condition.

Chronic sinusitis is, by definition, "an inflammation of the lining of the sinus cavities." These cavities occur over the eyes, beside the nose and in other areas of the body. Air pollution and overuse of antibiotics can cause inflammation, infection and even yeast overgrowth in these areas. The causes of the inflammation include stress, dry air, environmental or food allergies and dental problems. These areas should all be addressed, and then the mucous membranes must be allowed to heal and the immune system function strengthened. Humidifiers, saline nasal sprays (nonmedicated) and warm mists are helpful in soothing the mucous membrane lining. With central-heating and air-conditioning systems, humidity plunges extremely low, drying out the mucous membranes and making them more vulnerable to inflammation and infection. Increasing daily water intake to 64 ounces is recommended.

Dairy products should be avoided since they can cause inflammation and excess mucus production in some patients. Also avoid heavy exercise, which can weaken the immune system. Mild to moderate aerobic-type exercise is beneficial, however.

Echinacea and salt water

To stop the immediate problem of sinus inflammation, use steam and saline irrigation and brief courses of echinacea (three weeks on, one week off). Garlic should also be used daily (equivalent to one clove). I recommend 3,000–5,000 milligrams of vitamin C daily as well.

If these natural methods do not prove to be effective, I often recommend a minimally absorbable nasal anti-inflammatory spray such as Flonase for a short period of time, which can work wonders in many patients.

Many people complain of sinus problems that just won't go away. Actually many so-called sinus problems are really allergy problems. Secretions that build up in the sinus cavities and are not draining effectively usually cause true sinus problems (sinusitis), and these secretions can get infected.

There are some natural treatments and preventives that should be considered if excess mucus production, swelling and other chronic respiratory problems are present. Since most of these problems are due to allergies, it is important to understand that allergies are caused by an *overactive* immune system that stimulates enzymes. These enzymes, in turn, release histamine and other chemicals that cause the symptoms.

There are four natural substances, which block the enzymes causing the symptoms, that I suggest you try if you are battling this problem: carotenoids, fish oil, quercetin and resveratrol. Consider the brief explanation of each to help you decide how to use these helpful natural healers.

- Carotenoids: Typically found in yellow and orange foods, carotenoids should be increased not only in your diet but also in supplement form. They are cousins to beta carotene and include alpha carotene, lycopene, lutein and other mixed carotenoids. A daily supplement containing 2.5 milligrams of these various carotenoids is recommended.

- Fish oil: By now you should be familiar with the essential nutrients containing the omega-3 fatty acids found in many types of fish. A total of 600 milligrams should be consumed daily.

- Quercetin: Flavonoids are another type of potent antioxidant. Quercetin is a flavonoid that is particularly helpful for allergy/sinus problems. A daily dosage of 25 milligrams is recommended.

- Resveratrol: Found in the skin of red grapes, resveratrol is also an anti-inflammatory agent that can help relieve allergy or sinus symptoms.

Avoid dairy products

Excessive consumption of certain dairy products (particularly milk) can stimulate mucus production in many patients. Certain proteins in milk stimulate the formation of antibodies in the body, which can attack the mucous lining of the upper respiratory tract.

● ASK DR. CHERRY

QUESTION: Are there any negative side effects from taking echinacea?

ANSWER: Echinacea has been shown to have a stimulating effect on the immune system, but as I discussed earlier, stimulation is not always what our immune system needs. (See chapter 8.) So many of the diseases we see today are a result of the *overstimulation* of the immune system rather than an immune system that is understimulated. Echinacea can be helpful in small amounts when a person already has a cold or virus, but as I stated before, take it with care. If there is an underlying disease present that is caused by an overactive immune system—such as inflammatory bowel disease, asthma or arthritis—an "overdose" of echinacea can cause a full-fledged manifestation of the disease.

QUESTION: Can coming down with the flu cause any serious health problems?

ANSWER: Some recent studies have shown that the flu and other viruses can increase the future potential risk of Parkinson's disease. Some research has even indicated that the influenza-A virus may affect dopamine cells in the brain. A decrease in dopamine levels can result in Parkinson's disease years later.[1]

God has given us specific ways to strengthen and guard our bodies against these various viral attacks. We must do all we can to take care of our body, the temple of the Holy Spirit, using the knowledge we have to prevent unnecessary illness.

CHAPTER 10

DIABETES: STARVING IN THE LAND OF PLENTY

*Thus says the LORD, the God of David your
father: "I have heard your prayer, I have
seen your tears; surely I will heal you."*
—2 KINGS 20:5, NKJV

FATIGUE. BLINDNESS. DISFIGUREMENT DUE TO AMPUTATIONS. One devastating disease that affects millions of people is capable of wreaking havoc in the health and lives of those people upon whom it preys. You may not be aware that what actually occurs in a diabetic's body is starvation in the land of plenty. Even in the presence of nutrients, the cells of the body are unable to absorb what they need, resulting in multiple horrific symptoms.

Isn't it just like the devil to try to steal the provisions that God gives us, right from under our noses? In diabetes, he is literally "dangling a carrot" of glucose within millimeters of the cell wall, but because of the disease, the much-needed blood sugar is still just out of reach.

Diabetes is a disease that is reaching epidemic proportions in our society today. According to the Centers for Disease Control, approximately 17 million Americans suffer from the effects of diabetes, but one-third of these—almost 6.5 million people—don't even know that they have it![1]

Two thousand new cases of diabetes are diagnosed—not every month, not every week—but *every day.* Right now, diabetes has cost the American people over $100 billion—almost as much as the treatment costs for all forms of cancer. In the past eight years, diabetes has increased approximately 30 percent in the general population. However, among thirty-year-olds, type 2 diabetes—the most common type—has increased an incredible 70 percent.[2] Doctors and researchers used to call type 2 diabetes "adult-onset diabetes" because it very rarely struck anyone younger than the age of forty-five. But now, our definition is beginning to change because people as young as teenagers are developing glucose intolerance, which results in type 2 diabetes by the time they reach their twenties.

Why has diabetes become such an epidemic? Probably the biggest factor involved is the sedentary lifestyle of most Americans, which leads to weight gain. Over half of all Americans are now considered to be overweight, and this "extra baggage" is very harmful to their health. Specifically, being overweight causes the body to be less sensitive to the insulin it produces. In addition, the typical diet—high in saturated fats and sugars—that Americans consume is very conducive to the development of diabetes.

What Is Diabetes?

When a person eats a meal, the nutrients from the food are absorbed and enter the bloodstream to be carried to the cells of the body. *Glucose,* or blood sugar, is the primary molecule derived from food that passes through the walls of the blood vessels to reach the *receptor cells* of the muscle, nerves or other organs that need the blood sugar to function properly. The *pancreas* is the organ of the body that produces *insulin,* the primary substance that helps to transport the blood sugar into the cells of the body. As insulin is secreted by the pancreas into the bloodstream, the glucose levels in the blood are lowered as the blood sugar begins to pass through the walls of the blood vessels and into the receptor cells, which are waiting for nutrition.

Most people, following a fast, will have a glucose level of between 70 and 110—a normal level of glucose in the blood. But a diabetic's glucose level could reach 300. The unfortunate irony of this disease, however, is that despite the huge amount of sugar in the bloodstream, just out of reach of the receptor cells, the body is actually starving to death. Why? Because of something called *insulin resistance.*

Insulin resistance occurs because receptor cells, which have been exposed to too much insulin, become desensitized and are no longer able to absorb nutrients into the cells. In the beginning stages of diabetes, the pancreas still secretes normal levels of insulin, but as blood sugar rises, the body signals the pancreas to produce more insulin in order to get rid of the glut of sugar that is backing up in the bloodstream. The body is literally crying out, "More insulin over here, please!" since insulin is what transports sugar out of the blood into the cells.

Unfortunately, insulin levels that are either too high or too low will become a poison to the body. If insulin levels are too low, the body will starve because insulin is necessary for the absorption of nutrients. But when the pancreas begins to secrete more and more insulin into the bloodstream, the walls of the blood vessels are literally attacked with the substance. When this occurs in the coronary arteries or the vessels near the brain, risks of heart attack or stroke increase dramatically. In fact, 75 percent of my diabetic patients eventually die of a heart attack.

Spikes in insulin levels also decrease the sensitivity of the receptors to the point that they no longer function properly, and the cells can no longer absorb the nutrients that are "right outside of their grasp." Eventually, the pancreas wears itself out by overproducing so much insulin, and the person is forced to begin *insulin therapy.* Because their bodies no longer produce their own insulin, these people have to inject themselves with the insulin their body needs.

Many times, this problem of insulin resistance is compounded by our insatiable consumption of sugary junk foods. Just what happens when you eat that box of sugar doughnuts or indulge in that mid-afternoon Snickers bar? Shortly after the taste has faded from your mouth, your blood glucose level suddenly spikes as the sugar from the candy or the doughnut enters your bloodstream. Your body reacts by sending in a flux of insulin to counteract the glucose. These spikes in the insulin level are what decrease receptor sensitivity and create the insulin resistance. With certain types of sugar and junk food, the levels will first spike very high and then plummet very low, causing you to feel a burst of energy followed by fatigue and sluggishness.

The human body is designed to function best when there are gradual rises and declines in the glucose levels of the bloodstream. But our modern lifestyle, full of fast food that is overprocessed and sadly lacking in nutrition, serves to promote the development of diseases such as diabetes. In other words, the food that we eat is not only lacking in needed nutrition, but it is also killing us.

Symptoms of Diabetes

The following common symptoms of diabetes should be carefully noted, especially since diabetes consistently goes undiagnosed in people until it has progressed to dangerous phases:

- *Increased thirst.* When the body is facing an unusual amount of glucose in the bloodstream, it calls upon the kidneys to help get rid of the glut. In order to dilute the glucose, the kidneys begin to excrete fluid, which increases the need for fluid, hence, increased thirst. Accompanying this symptom is *increased urination,* the kidneys' attempt to flush the bloodstream of the excess glucose.

- *Fatigue.* As the disease progresses, although there is more than adequate nutrition in the blood, the cells are not receiving it due to insulin resistance, as I explained. For this reason most diabetics complain of feeling totally exhausted. Ironically, they have the highest fuel supply in their bloodstream (300–400 glucose levels), but their cells are literally starving to death.

- *Weight loss.* As the body continues to starve, it will begin to feed on its stores of fat and muscle, and the person will begin to lose weight.

- *Blurred vision.* As sugar levels in the blood continue to rise, the blood vessels in the eyes will begin to be adversely affected. If left unchecked, diabetes will lead to partial or complete *blindness.* In fact, diabetes is one of the leading causes of blindness.

- *Neuropathy.* Every nerve in the body is connected to a blood vessel in order to receive life-giving nutrients, which means that every nerve in the body is affected by the high glucose levels of diabetes. As the disease progresses, the person will notice tingling in the extremities as nerves become damaged, a condition known as neuropathy. Advanced *peripheral neuropathy* affects extremities, leading to increased lack of feeling in the arms and legs and potentially dangerous sores, which go unnoticed by the person, leading to infections or even gangrene. Often amputation becomes the necessary drastic measure that must be taken to save the patient's life. Advanced *autonomic neuropathy* affects internal organs of the body like nerves to the stomach, making the patient unable to digest food properly, or nerves to the male genitalia, making the person impotent.

⮑ *Kidney failure.* Finally, because the kidneys work so hard to remove excess glucose from the blood, the incidence of renal disease, kidney failure and dialysis increase dramatically in the diabetic population.

Diagnosing Diabetes

I cannot emphasize enough how important it is for you, if you are experiencing any of these symptoms, to go to your doctor right away to have your blood sugar levels tested. It is easy to overlook the symptoms and pretend that nothing is wrong. A few years ago, I saw a patient who thought he had found a new way to lose weight by drinking lots of water. He did not realize that both his weight loss and his thirst were classic symptoms of diabetes. When I performed a blood test on him, we discovered that his glucose level was over 350!

Be aware of the wiles of the devil; he would love to take out as many members of the body of Christ as he can with this deadly disease. If you have any of the symptoms of diabetes, be sure to consult with your physician immediately. He can perform simple tests to determine whether you are struggling with diabetes.

Glycosylated hemoglobin test

This test is more simply known as the Hemoglobin A1c. Its advantage over several others is that it averages a person's blood sugar levels over a time period of three months, instead of just taking a random sampling here and there. This is important because a true diabetic's numbers can vary drastically from day to day.

The goal of the A1c test is one simple number: Keep the A1c under seven, and you will be all right.

Glucose tolerance test (GTT)

This test requires the patient to take 75 grams of glucose and have their blood levels tested two hours later. Problems occur when this number reaches the level of 150 to 200.

Fasting blood sugar test

If a blood sugar level, after a twelve-hour fast, reaches 126 or higher on two or more different days, by definition, the patient is diagnosed as having diabetes.

Conventional Treatments for Diabetes

Many Christians resist the idea of taking medication for a disease or illness, but if you need to be on a prescription medicine or insulin treatment for diabetes, it may save your life. There are several natural treatments for the disease, which I will discuss later in this chapter. But most of the prescription drugs that are available for diabetes are much more effective at lowering the patient's blood sugar levels *quickly* and *predictably*.

If you are just discovering that you are a diabetic, chances are that you need to lower your glucose levels, and you need to lower them *fast*. Often the best plan, the plan that God guides many people to take, is to begin to take the prescription medicine immediately, but also to begin taking natural supplements at the same time. Many times when the glucose levels are stabilized, the patient can begin to back off some of the prescriptions. But I cannot emphasize enough that *any changes that you make must be made under a doctor's supervision and while your blood levels are being monitored.* Diabetes is a dangerous disease; don't allow the enemy to get a foothold in your life by ignoring wisdom and prudence. Allow your doctor to be an instrument of God's healing in your life.

Medications to treat diabetes have classically addressed the diminishing levels of insulin in the bloodstream. Glucotrol is one among several of these drugs that stimulate the pancreas to secrete more insulin, but this is not an ideal solution to the problem. Certainly, diabetics whose insulin levels are too low will need a way either to produce more insulin within their own bodies or to receive shots of insulin that are injected directly into their bloodstream. However, increasing insulin levels simply to counteract increasing glucose levels in the blood does not address the root of the problem, and, as I mentioned before, too much insulin is very harmful to the body.

Another class of drugs used to treat diabetes actually reduces the insulin resistance of the cells. Remember, insulin resistance occurs when cell receptors that have been exposed to too much insulin become desensitized and are no longer able to absorb nutrients from the bloodstream into the cells.

Doctors are beginning to realize that if a patient's pancreas is still able to produce a normal level of insulin, perhaps a better strategy for treatment would be to cause the receptor cells to become more sensitive to the insulin that is already available.

A third class of prescription drugs is just beginning to show promise in the treatment of diabetes. These drugs affect the breakdown of carbohydrates in the system, slowing them down, which in turn prevents the extreme glucose spikes in the bloodstream. Both glucose and insulin levels remain steady, and diabetic symptoms are brought under control. Precose is one of these drugs that are showing promise in this form of treatment.

Natural Nutrients to Prevent or Reverse Diabetes

I am so thankful to God that He has provided natural resources for healing. Many substances available in the plant and animal kingdoms very nearly duplicate the same effects of prescription medications used to treat diabetes. If you have diabetes, or if diabetes runs in your family, begin taking these nutrients *now* to begin slowing the progression of your disease or, better still, prevent or reverse it.

Chromium

Chromium is a natural trace mineral that should be present in our daily diets, but the majority of Americans are chromium deficient. Most of us consume only 30 micrograms of chromium a day, when we need 200 micrograms daily.

In the treatment of diabetes, chromium actually increases the effectiveness of insulin. That is, in the presence of chromium, the insulin produced in the pancreas actually does a better job of moving the glucose through the blood vessels and to the receptor cells.

Chromium can be found naturally in brewer's yeast, which is available at your local health food store. However, that may still not give you a sufficient amount daily. I recommend a chromium supplement of 300 micrograms a day for the *prevention* of diabetes and 800 to 1000 micrograms a day for the *treatment* of the disease.

Vanadium

The trace element vanadium is also effective in enhancing the effect of the insulin already present in the body. Vanadium itself has insulin-like properties, which cause blood sugar levels to drop. The same dosage of 300 micrograms daily is recommended for both preventive and treatment purposes.

Biotin

Biotin, one of the B vitamins, operates in much the same way as the third class of prescription medicines we discussed previously: It enhances the metabolism or the breakdown of carbohydrates, reducing the number of glucose spikes in the bloodstream. The ideal dosage for biotin is also 300 micrograms daily.

Niacin

Niacin performs the same function as biotin; that is, it increases carbohydrate metabolism. The dosage of niacin should be carefully monitored and kept to a maximum of 100 milligrams daily; this should help to prevent any adverse effects to the liver.

Magnesium

Many Americans are deficient in magnesium; the recommended daily dosage is 400 milligrams per day. Magnesium has numerous beneficial effects in the treatment of diabetes. First of all, it causes an increase in the excretion of glucose in the urine, thus helping to alleviate some of the excess blood sugars that a diabetic experiences. Magnesium, like biotin and niacin, also improves carbohydrate metabolism. And finally, magnesium increases the cellular sensitivity to insulin, diminishing insulin resistance, which is the greatest problem that the majority of diabetics face.

Zinc

Again, most of our diets are deficient in the levels of zinc that we need. A 15-milligram daily dose is needed for the prevention and treatment of diabetes, but this is another nutrient that should be approached with caution. Some people think that if 15 milligrams are good, then ten times that would be even better. That is incorrect! Too much zinc will adversely affect the metabolism of both glucose and insulin, so please be sure to take only 15 milligrams per day.

Omega-3 fatty acids

God's provision made nutrients available to us in both the plant and animal kingdoms. The omega-3 fatty acids are found in the animal kingdom, in the fatty fishes such as salmon, cod, mackerel or herring. These fatty acids have been shown both to improve glucose breakdown and to decrease the body's resistance to insulin.

Herbal Preparations to Combat Diabetes

In addition to the seven essential nutrients listed above, there are four herbal preparations that are effective in combating diabetes and in controlling some of its complications. When used together, these nutrients and herbs have a *synergistic* effect, working together to become even more effective in bringing health to your body.

Gymnema

This important herb with the unusual name is from a woody plant that grows in India and in the Far East. It has been used for centuries in the treatment of diabetes. Numerous benefits can be derived from the consumption of gymnema: It decreases blood sugar levels; it decreases insulin requirements; it regenerates the beta cells of the pancreas and allows them to produce more insulin; and it aids the glucose in crossing the blood vessel wall to reach nutritionally deprived cells.

Many patients have been able to reduce or phase out their prescription medications after a regimen of gymnema. It is now sold at health food stores and should be taken in a dosage of 400 milligrams per day.

Bitter melon

Bitter melon, like gymnema, has the effect of increasing glucose uptake (absorption) into the cells. It comes in an extract form and should be taken at a dose of 100 to 200 milligrams, three times a day.

Fenugreek

Fenugreek, another herb with an unusual name, works differently in that it stops the absorption of sugar in the patient's gastrointestinal tract, thus lowering the glucose levels that reach the bloodstream. Fenugreek is the fiber portion of a certain herbal seed. It should be taken at a dosage of 15 to 25 grams per day.

Bilberry

Bilberry, or bilberry extract, prevents capillaries and blood vessels from leakage, a common problem among diabetics. Two hundred milligrams per day is the recommended dosage.

Counteracting Complications of Diabetes

Perhaps the most frightening aspect of diabetes lies in the numerous harrowing complications that could potentially occur: blindness, heart attacks, strokes, disfigurement or even amputation of the extremities, along with damage to internal organs. These complications may at first seem to be diverse, but they all stem from the same general problem: *neuropathy*. (See page 85 for explanation.) There are three important natural substances that can help prevent serious complications of diabetes.

Alpha lipoic acid

Alpha lipoic acid is produced in very small amounts in the human body, which is why it is not classified as a vitamin per se. When taken at a supplemental dose of 50 milligrams per day, it improves the metabolism of sugar, increases muscular energy, regenerates other powerful antioxidants such as vitamins C, E and glutathione, and it protects against the possibility of neuropathy. However, if you are already suffering the effects of neuropathy, the suggested dose increases to 600 to 800 milligrams per day, depending on the severity of your symptoms. The good news is that alpha lipoic acid has no known side effects.

GLA: Gamma linolenic acid

GLA is an essential fatty acid, a cousin of the omega-3 fish oils, which we have already discussed. Dosage, for prevention and treatment, is 90 milligrams per day.

Water-soluble B vitamins

Water-soluble B vitamins, including B_1, B_6, B_{12}, inositol and B_5, increase nerve sheath conduction. When this takes place in the brain, the result is improved memory function, but the benefits can be reaped throughout the body. Water-soluble B vitamins nourish the nerves and supply damaged nerves with blood, preventing infection and gangrene in extremities, as well as other complications.

Daily Regimen to Prevent Diabetes

Neither my wife nor I have diabetes, but we do certain things every day to ensure that we never contract this deadly disease. I have listed below the six most important prevention techniques for diabetes. These techniques take self-discipline to implement in your life, but the results are worth the effort.

1. Take the three most important minerals daily.

These include the daily dosages of chromium, vanadium and magnesium. Because so many of our diets are deficient in these minerals, I recommend taking them in supplement form. These three will make your own body's insulin more effective and decrease your cell's insulin resistance.

2. Take the daily dose of the antioxidants alpha lipoic acid and lycopene.

Alpha lipoic acid and lycopene are the most powerful antioxidants against the effects of diabetes. By taking a supplement of just 50 milligrams a day of alpha lipoic acid and 1,000 micrograms a day of lycopene, your blood insulin levels can be decreased significantly.

3. Take the essential fatty acids, including fish oil and GLA.

Omega-3 fatty acids (fish oil) and GLA are effective in preventing diabetes by improving glucose tolerance.

4. Watch your diet.

Cut back on the sugary junk food that causes your glucose levels to spike and then plummet. Adding the following nutrients to your diet will help immensely:

- Two servings a day of a whole-grain food product (dark rice; dark, crunchy bread; or a grainy cereal) will decrease the risk of diabetes by 33 percent.[3] One of the best cereals we have found for this purpose is called Bran Buds, made by Kellogg's.

- Psyllium is a fiber extract from the husk of the plantago plant, which can also be found in Bran Buds. It has been found to decrease blood sugar levels by 11 percent in people who consumed 2 tablespoons per day. In these same people, it decreased the post-meal sugar levels (the dangerous glucose spikes) by 20 percent.[4]

- In addition to the chromium supplements you should already be taking, it's a good idea to add to your diet foods that are high in chromium. These include asparagus, mushrooms, almonds and prunes.

- Other foods that can prevent diabetes include onions, which contain diphenylamine, a compound that can decrease blood sugar levels as effectively as a prescription drug; cinnamon, which lowers blood sugar and increases cellular sensitivity to insulin; and beans, which slow the rise of glucose in the blood stream. Who would have thought that such common foods, which most of us already have in our pantries, can help prevent one of the most deadly diseases in our society?

5. Exercise.

Check with your doctor before beginning any exercise program, but make sure that you work some form of regular exercise—whether it be walking, jogging or playing tennis—into your lifestyle. Regular exercise can dramatically reduce the risk of diabetes.

6. Lose weight.

If you regularly follow steps one through five, you will lose weight as well. Obesity is a growing problem in America. Dropping the pounds will greatly decrease your risk for diabetes.

ASK DR. CHERRY

QUESTION: **If I have just been diagnosed with diabetes, why shouldn't I just start immediately taking the natural substances that you have recommended?**

ANSWER: If your diabetes has just been diagnosed and you have not received any other treatment for the disease, it is possible that your blood sugar levels are dangerously high. You may need to take one of the available prescription medications to bring both your glucose and your insulin levels back under control. Of course, you should also begin a simultaneous treatment regimen of the natural substances I have discussed. Many of my patients are eventually able to phase out their prescription medications once they have been taking the natural substances for a period of time. Be sure that you have your doctor monitor your blood levels during this critical period so that your health is maintained and you don't inadvertently cause any medical crises.

QUESTION: **How important is it to follow the six steps to prevent diabetes if the disease does not run in my family?**

ANSWER: As I stated before, neither my wife, Linda, nor I show any symptoms of developing the disease, but we follow the six prevention steps diligently. Again, implementing these steps into your life takes a great deal of discipline. You may have the best of intentions, but also have a craving for doughnuts! The Bible says that it is the spirit of a man that sustains him in his infirmity (Prov. 18:14). Put your body in subjection to your own spirit and to what the Spirit of God is telling you to do. Remind yourself of the benefits these steps will have for your total well-being—not just in the prevention of diabetes—and that you are more than a conqueror in Christ!

ESSENTIAL NUTRIENTS TO MAINTAIN HEALTHY GLUCOSE LEVELS

NUTRIENT	EFFECT	PREVENTIVE DOSAGE	TREATMENT DOSAGE
Alpha lipoic acid	Improves sugar metabolism; regenerates other antioxidants	50 mg	600–800 mg
Bitter melon fruit extract	Herb shown in both human and animal studies to have a beneficial effect on blood glucose levels[5]	400 mg	600 mg
Bilberry leaf extract	Herb used in traditional folk medicine to treat diabetes and its complications	200 mg	200 mg
Chromium	Essential trace mineral that plays a role in glucose regulation and helps increase the effectiveness of insulin	300 mcg	800–1,000 mcg
Fenugreek	Soluble fiber that slows the absorption of sugars from the intestinal tract; binds toxins; helps regulate cholesterol levels	15–25 grams	15–25 grams
Gymnema leaf extract	Unique herb from India that has been shown to lower insulin requirements in clinical studies, possibly by helping to regenerate the insulin-producing cells of the pancreas[6]	400 mg	400 mg
Magnesium	Essential mineral needed for proper insulin function; often deficient in diabetics	400 mg	400 mg
Vanadium	Trace mineral known to support insulin function and improve glucose utilization	300 mcg	300 mcg
Biotin	B vitamin that enhances the metabolism of carbohydrates	300 mcg	300 mcg
Niacin	Vitamin that enhances the metabolism of carbohydrates	100 mg	100 mg
Gamma linolenic acid	Improves glucose breakdown and decreases resistance to insulin	90 mg	90 mg

CHAPTER 11

NUTRITION &
GASTROINTESTINAL
DISORDERS

*Worship the LORD your God, and his blessing will
be on your food and water. I will take away sickness from among you, and none will miscarry or be
barren in your land. I will give you a full life span.*
—EXODUS 23:25–26, NIV

Y OU ARE WHAT YOU EAT. When you were growing up, did you ever
hear this statement? Perhaps your mother made this declaration as
she was trying to get you to finish the vegetables on your plate. But was
she right? To a certain degree, she was, but a more accurate way to put it
would be, "You are what you eat *and* what you are able to absorb." You
can eat all the lima beans and green peas in the world, but unless your body
can absorb the nutrients in these vegetables, they don't do you any good!

Like many other diseases in our culture, gastrointestinal disorders are on
the rise. From ailments as common as heartburn to more serious problems
such as ulcers, acid reflux disease and irritable bowel syndrome, your digestive system is under attack. In a manner similar to the immune system, the
digestive system is your first line of defense against harmful agents in the
world around you. All the nutrients your body takes in pass through the
digestive system. It is therefore crucial to maintain gastrointestinal health
and protect your body from attack in this area.

Four Processes of Digestion

When you consider the digestive system, you may sensibly conclude that its primary function is to digest food. That is true to an extent, but the digestive system does much more than that for the body. There are four major processes of digestion that will be helpful to understand for protecting your health:

1. Your body must *digest* food. Obviously, you must take in the food and begin to break it down into various tiny components that the body can use for energy.

2. Your body must *eliminate* waste. Not every molecule of food that you take in can be used by the body, so what is not helpful or good for you must be sorted out and then removed.

3. Your body must *absorb* nutrients. As I mentioned at the beginning of the chapter, you can eat all the food you can fit into your stomach, but if you cannot absorb the nutrition available in that food, you will literally starve to death.

4. Your body must *normalize* its balance of "good" bacteria in your intestines. Otherwise known as *flora,* these "good" bacteria must be present in the colon for your body to function properly.

I like to call these four processes the "D-E-A-N" of digestion:

∾ D-igest

∾ E-liminate

∾ A-bsorb

∾ N-ormalize

All four processes must be operating successfully to prevent or treat gastrointestinal disorders.

The Importance of Enzymes

When you ingest food into your body, digestion begins almost immediately. *Digestion* essentially means the breakdown of food into a form that can be absorbed by the body, and it cannot take place except in the presence of *enzymes*. There are many types of enzymes in the body, but for our purposes, we will examine key enzymes that are crucial to maintain your digestive health. These include the *amylase* enzymes, the *lipase* enzymes and the *proteases* or *proteolytic* enzymes.

- Amylase enzymes break down carbohydrates.
- Lipase enzymes break down fats.
- Proteolytic enzymes break down proteins.

Through the work of these three types of enzymes, the entire gamut of nutrients available in the four major food groups are available to us. Lactase, an amylase enzyme, is necessary to break down the lactose that is found in milk. Some people do not produce this enzyme and are therefore lactose intolerant, or unable to drink milk without experiencing discomfort such as gas or bloating. Cellulase is another important amylase enzyme; it breaks down various vegetables that we eat.

Although they are produced in smaller amounts in various parts of the digestive tract, these enzymes are primarily secreted by the *pancreas*. The more enzymes the pancreas has to produce, the more it can be subjected to stress and fatigue. Therefore, one of the first steps to take to ensure the health of the digestive system is to supplement these primary enzymes as a part of your daily diet. Two hundred milligrams each should be taken daily of amylase, cellulase, lactase, lipase and the protease enzymes.

Enzyme Deficiency

A deficiency in any of these enzymes can result in a host of uncomfortable digestive problems: gas, bloating, diarrhea or constipation. Without the proper amounts of enzymes necessary for digestion to take place, particles of food will pass through the body, undigested, and create these difficulties. A more serious effect, however, of an enzyme deficiency is fatigue. If problems are occurring at the digestive stage of the process, the food that is eaten is not broken down to a stage where it is absorbable by the body; therefore, the cells will not be receiving the nutrition that they need. Energy sources are quickly depleted, and you feel tired all the time.

One unusual ailment that is in early stages of research is called the *leaky gut syndrome*. This occurs when the proteolytic enzymes (protein digestion) are either not present in sufficient quantities or they are not functioning correctly. Leaky gut syndrome is believed to take place when larger protein molecules that have missed being properly digested migrate to the "gut," or small intestine, and are absorbed there rather than earlier in the digestive tract as God intended. This absorption in an inappropriate area creates an immunological response from the body, and it could be a cause of such immune-related problems as allergies or arthritis.

Konjac Root: Digestive Helper

The body cannot use everything you eat, so the "leftovers" must be eliminated. You have no doubt heard that it is important to eat more fiber. That is because fiber helps in this elimination process. The fibers that are most helpful are water soluble; this means they are able to absorb the water from the waste product. The konjac root, common to Japan and widely used by the Japanese, may contribute significantly to their health, giving them the longest average life span of any other people in the world.

From the konjac root an unusual water-soluble fiber called glucomannan is formulated. The most amazing aspect about glucomannan is the sheer amount of water it can absorb: *two hundred times* its own weight in water! That means that very small amounts of it can have a big effect in absorbing watery waste in our intestines. Another significant aspect of glucomannan is that it aids in the absorption of cholesterol, all the while creating a feeling of fullness in the stomach, as it soaks up water and expands. It contains no calories and suppresses the appetite because of its volume. For these reasons, the konjac root is becoming important as a weight loss supplement.

Another important function of glucomannan is its ability to regulate blood sugar. Through its immediate absorption of water, it slows down the absorption of sugar into the bloodstream; it can therefore be essential in leveling out the spikes and drops in blood sugar that are so harmful, especially to diabetics.

Yet another benefit of the konjac root is that it counters constipation. Glucomannan, after soaking up so much water, contains a fairly large water volume. As it passes through the intestines, it mixes with the stool and actually acts as a stool softener to prevent hard stools and constipation.

Water-soluble fibers, such as pectin or oat bran, will perform most of these functions, but the difference with the konjac root is that a very *small amount of glucomannan produces very big results!* I recommend 400 milligrams of glucomannan daily. With other fibers, people have to drink large glasses of fiber solutions that taste terrible in order to get the benefits that the concentrated levels in the konjac root provide with just a tiny amount. And because the amount is so small, it can be put inside of a capsule that can be swallowed and dissolved in the stomach. That's good news for a lot of people!

Did You Say "*Good* Bacteria"?

While problems in enzyme production will affect the digestive functions of the body, other potential difficulties can occur when the balance between "good" and "bad" bacteria in the intestines is disrupted. It seems strange to some people that any sort of bacteria could be beneficial, but it is true. God created these good bacteria, or flora, to live in our intestines and overwhelm the bad bacteria that could cause infections or other serious illnesses. There are over four hundred different species of helpful flora naturally residing in the colon, two of the most common being *bifidobacterium* and *lactobacillus*.

One of the most interesting terms used to describe this type of bacteria is *probiotic*. When you consider the literal meaning of that word, it has special significance to us as Christians who understand that God created our bodies to be the temple, or dwelling place, for His Holy Spirit. *Probiotic* means "pro life," or "promoting life." When, for instance, you inadvertently drink polluted water that contains harmful bacteria, the probiotic bacteria in your digestive systems go to work and attack the foreign invader, literally promoting life in your body.

Another function of the flora is to keep the normal yeast levels of the intestines in balance. If this gets out of hand, especially in women, commonly recurring yeast infections will take place. An underlying cause of these infections is an insufficient amount of good bacteria in the colon. Additionally, some forms of bacteria in the intestines assist in the production of enzymes, one of which is lactase, the enzyme discussed earlier that breaks down the lactose sugars in milk and dairy products. One potential cause, then, of lactose intolerance could be a deficiency in the bacteria that produce lactase.

Why Antibiotics Can Actually Be Harmful

Again, the common misconception that most people have is that all bacteria are bad, and therefore all antibiotics must be good. But take into account our definition of the probiotic bacteria: If *probiotic* means to promote life, then what might *antibiotic* mean? Yes, antibiotics are literally "against life," most commonly against the life of bad bacteria, but when you ingest an antibiotic into your body, it doesn't know the difference between good bacteria and bad bacteria. It kills them all.

Sometimes a round of antibiotics is necessary to knock out a bacterial infection or a case of pneumonia, but I must emphasize that if you have taken antibiotics for whatever reason, you must recolonize your intestines with the good flora that were wiped out by the antibiotics.

The following substances may be taken to restore a normal balance of bacteria in the intestines:

- Arabinogalactan, 250 milligrams per day
- Fructooligosaccharides, 100 milligrams per day
- Lactobacillus, 150 milligrams per day

You may be saying to yourself, "I haven't needed to take an antibiotic for years!" Even if that is the case, it is a good idea to recolonize your intestines periodically. You may not have been prescribed an antibiotic by your doctor, but have you eaten chicken lately? Poultry, among other animals raised for our food supply, are regularly treated with antibiotics, which remain in their system right up until the time we take that first bite. And every bite thereafter is slowly killing off the good bacteria in your colon.

For these reasons, it is important for all of us to supplement our digestive system with probiotics, enzymes and the fiber found in the konjac root. Begin to add these things to your diet, and watch God begin to restore your digestive health.

ASK DR. CHERRY

QUESTION: **I have heard about something called colon cleansing, which seems to be gaining popularity. Does that work?**

ANSWER: Colon cleansing has been a fad that has been gaining in popularity the last fifteen years or so. And again, it is based partially on the mistaken belief that "all bacteria are bad," and so it would be good for the body to wash as much bacteria out of it as possible. Some people mistakenly get excited over colon irrigation, but what they don't realize is that they are stripping their colon clean of the flora that it needs and leaving it defenseless against the bad bacteria that will inevitably come back on the scene.

What I suggest to many people is that by adding the good bacteria back into the colon, these bacteria will reproduce themselves and attack the bad bacteria for you. You don't have to go through the discomfort of a colon cleansing to destroy the harmful agents in your intestines. Isn't God good?

One good way He has given us to restore this good bacteria is by eating yogurt—not the frozen kind, but the "slimy" yogurt because it is what contains the bacteria that are good for you. Some of us, like my wife, Linda, don't like yogurt; if that is the case, it is possible to restore the flora through a supplement, which has no taste.

QUESTION: **What is diverticulitis, and what can be done to prevent it?**

ANSWER: Diverticulosis is a condition in which excess pressure builds up inside of the colon, usually caused by constipation or hard stool. When the condition progresses to the stage in which inflammation occurs, it becomes diverticulitis. The best way to prevent this painful and problematic illness is to soften the stools and keep them regular by adding fiber to the diet. Eating oatmeal or Kellogg's Bran Buds cereal each morning is a good way to accomplish this, as it contains two different fibers and has been shown effective in maintaining stool regularity. Another good idea is to avoid small seeds, popcorn hulls or anything small and indigestible that could cause further irritation along the wall of the colon.

Essential Nutrients to Keep Your System on Track

NUTRIENT	EFFECT	DAILY DOSAGE
Amylase	Enzyme that helps in the digestion of carbohydrates	200 mg
Cellulase	Enzyme that helps in the digestion of cellulose, a fiber found in many fruits and vegetables	200 mg
Lactase	Enzyme that improves the digestion of lactose (milk sugar)	200 mg
Lipase	Enzyme that helps in the digestion of fats	200 mg
Protease I	Enzyme that helps in the digestion of meat proteins and helps reduce inflammation	200 mg
Protease II	Enzyme that helps in the digestion of plant proteins and helps reduce inflammation	200 mg
Protease III	Enzyme that helps in the digestion of milk proteins and helps reduce inflammation	200 mg
Glucomannan	Natural source of soluble fiber that helps eliminate toxins, enhance healthy blood sugar levels, reduce bloating, improve stool transit time and stool weight, support healthy cholesterol and fat metabolism, and create bulk for healthy regularity and elimination	400 mg
Arabinogalactan	Fiber-like substance that promotes the growth of friendly bacteria in the gut while suppressing the growth of harmful organisms	250 mg
Fructooligo-saccharides	Fiber-like substance that helps reduce bad bacteria while supporting friendly bacteria	100 mg
Lactobacillus sporogenes	Beneficial intestinal organism that reduces population of harmful organisms	150 mg

CHAPTER 12

TREAT ACID REFLUX DISEASE NATURALLY

*And Jesus went about all Galilee, teaching in their
synagogues, preaching the gospel of the kingdom,
and healing all kinds of sickness and all kinds
of disease among the people.*
—MATTHEW 4:23, NKJV

MUST HAVE BEEN THE PIZZA." You groan as you toss and turn in your bed. Heartburn has struck again, and you can kiss your hope for a restful night's sleep good-bye.

Periodic episodes of heartburn caused by acid reflux are very common. However, when these episodes occur frequently, they can become much more than just a nuisance. In fact, frequent episodes of acid reflux (technically known as *gastroesophageal reflux disease,* or GERD) can increase the potential risk of esophageal cancer by causing changes in the cells lining the esophagus.

Five Ways to Quench Heartburn

Here are five helpful suggestions that have been proven to quench heartburn—without the use of prescription medicine. They are simple at-home techniques that I would recommend you try before seeking help from your doctor. However, if you are consistently experiencing more than three episodes of heartburn a week, you should see your doctor as soon as possible to help prevent developing scar tissue in your esophagus.

1. Eat large meals early and light meals later.

Years ago people tended to eat larger meals in the early part of the day and lighter meals in the evening. Now the typical pattern is reversed. Many people skip breakfast, eat a small lunch and consume their largest meal in the evening. This is just the opposite of the way God designed our bodies to function. At the same time our eating patterns changed, the degree of obesity increased. The combination of these factors has produced increasing problems with esophageal disease.

There is a muscular valve known as a *sphincter* between the esophagus and the stomach. The lining of the stomach is designed to handle a high acid level, but if this acid "refluxes," or backs up, into the esophagus, problems can occur. The cells lining the esophagus are not designed to handle high acid levels. The acid can cause severe damage and even erosions and inflammation in the esophagus that can produce the symptoms of heartburn.

When you eat late in the evening, large amounts of food are in the stomach when you lie down at night, producing pressure on the muscular sphincter. If you are carrying extra pounds, it produces additional pressure on the stomach, which in turn causes more acid to enter the esophagus. The simple habit of eating a light meal early in the evening can dramatically reduce the symptoms of reflux.

2. Raise the head of your bed.

By placing a small block of wood such as a 2 x 4 (or even a 4 x 4 block, in some cases) under the head of the bed, you can elevate the entire bed. This prevents the return of acid into the esophagus and helps contain the acid in the stomach where it belongs. Adding an extra pillow or two under your head can actually make the problem worse because of the angle created between the esophagus and the stomach.

3. Avoid the three "bad guys": peppermint candy, coffee and chocolate.

There are certain substances that can weaken the tone or strength of the sphincter muscle, allowing acid to reflux. These include coffee, peppermint candy and chocolate. Isn't it ironic that many times after a meal at a restaurant, we have a cup of coffee, a peppermint candy or a chocolate mint?

4. Drink more water.

A simple remedy for heartburn that has proven effective is to increase your daily consumption of water. The water tends to wash the acid off the wall of the esophagus.

5. Use antacids with caution.

If you need to use an occasional antacid, remember that the liquid antacids are better than the tablets because they tend to adhere to the esophagus, forming a protective coating. There are over-the-counter medications known as H2 blockers, which include Tagamet and similar medications. These can be used on occasion, but as we get older, the stomach tends to produce less acid, and the chronic use of these medications to neutralize acid can sometimes interfere with digestion.

 ASK DR. CHERRY

QUESTION: **How do I know whether the pain I feel in my chest is heartburn or a more serious cardiac problem?**

ANSWER: Sometimes it is difficult to tell what the root cause of a certain pain actually is. Many times, a burning sensation of pain in the chest is heartburn that is due to acid in the esophagus, but sometimes heartburn can be caused by an underlying problem with the heart. Or the pain could be cardiovascular in nature, but have nothing to do with heartburn. Because it is so difficult to tell the difference between these types of pain, if you have any doubts, be sure to check with your doctor.

QUESTION: **When does heartburn become more than just a nuisance and constitute a serious problem for which I should seek help?**

ANSWER: If you are consistently having more than three episodes of heartburn weekly, you should get additional information from your own physician. Don't allow these symptoms to continue long term. I have seen patients who have ignored the problem, hoping it would just go away. Instead, they had developed scar tissue in their esophagus. The scar tissue narrows the esophagus, which obviously can cause major difficulties and even require surgical correction.

On occasion, God has directed me to use with a patient the most potent medication known for acid reflux disease—proton pump inhibitors. None of us like to take prescription medication, but God can and does use these medicines to protect us from the dire consequences of severe acid reflux disease.

CHAPTER 13

NATURAL RELIEF FOR IRRITABLE BOWEL SYNDROME

Great multitudes followed Him [Jesus],
and He healed them all.
—MATTHEW 12:15, NKJV

T HIS UNPLEASANT SYNDROME AFFECTS MILLIONS OF PEOPLE. Irritable bowel syndrome (formerly known as spastic colon) can be a very frustrating and troublesome syndrome. This has been one of the most frustrating disorders facing the medical profession. In fact, it is the number-one referral made by family physicians to GI specialists (gastroenterologists).

Irritable bowel syndrome—not to be confused with inflammatory bowel disease, such as ulcerative colitis or Crohn's disease—affects millions of people. The exact cause is still not fully understood, but it appears to be a problem with the transmission of nerve impulses affecting the nerve endings to the smooth muscles in the GI tract. We also know that it has been associated with periods of high stress. Symptoms include abdominal bloating and cramping, excessive gas and either diarrhea or constipation or alternating between the two.

Peppermint Oil

An effective natural treatment for irritable bowel syndrome is enteric-coated peppermint oil. Research has indicated that the oil found in the peppermint plant can relax smooth muscles in the colon. Prescription muscle relaxants (known as *antispasmodics*) can cause numerous side effects, but the peppermint oil found in the plant kingdom has no side effects.[1]

There is one small problem with peppermint oil, however. In the last chapter we listed peppermint as a major irritant of acid reflux. If you have acid reflux disease as well as irritable bowel syndrome, it is imperative that you take the coated capsule form of the peppermint oil so that the oil will be absorbed in the intestine rather than in the stomach.

Excellent results have been seen with the use of peppermint oil. It tends to stop the excessive spasms in the smooth muscles and helps maintain the muscle tone in the colon. Peppermint oil capsules have been used for several years in Europe for the treatment of irritable bowel syndrome and have been found to be very safe and effective.

Researchers in Britain have recorded a nearly 50 percent reduction in colon spasms after peppermint oil was introduced into the colon. The capsules are available in a standardized, coated form that contains 0.2 milliliters of peppermint oil. One to two capsules daily between meals were used in the study. Peppermint must be taken properly to avoid the complications associated with acid reflux disease, as I mentioned earlier.[2]

Other Treatments for Irritable Bowel Syndrome

Believe me, if you are suffering from severe symptoms of irritable bowel syndrome, you want *relief*. Sometimes a safe prescription medication may be required to relax the smooth muscle. Smooth muscle relaxants that have been proven effective include dicyclomine, cimetropium, mebeverine and trimebutine. These agents prove to be very effective for relieving the abdominal pain and discomfort of irritable bowel syndrome. At least thirteen out of sixteen studies showed an improvement in symptoms while patients were on these medications.[3]

Other traditional treatments for irritable bowel syndrome include psyllium and wheat bran, although these are not as effective and can cause gas in quite a few patients.

If peppermint oil capsules do not relieve the symptoms, try adding very small amounts of wheat bran. (An ideal amount would be ¼ cup of Kellogg's Bran Buds cereal.)

ASK DR. CHERRY

QUESTION: **What causes irritable bowel syndrome?**

ANSWER: Like so many other health conditions, irritable bowel syndrome has multiple causes. Food allergies, excessive stress, altered bacterial flora in the intestinal tract and a lack of fiber in the diet are all thought to be contributors to irritable bowel syndrome.

QUESTION: **What is the difference between irritable bowel syndrome and inflammatory bowel disease?**

ANSWER: Both irritable bowel syndrome (IBS) and inflammatory bowel disease (IBD) can cause considerable discomfort and pain, not to mention emotional distress, in the patients they affect. Both have similar symptoms such as abdominal bloating, cramping, excessive gas and diarrhea. However, inflammatory bowel *disease,* which includes colitis and Crohn's disease, is more serious, as patients usually begin to pass blood in the stool. IBS has its root cause in the muscles of the colon, which spasm uncontrollably. However, IBD appears to be an autoimmune disorder, in which the body's own defense systems attack itself.

QUESTION: **After diagnosing my problem as irritable bowel syndrome, my gastroenterologist prescribed an antidepressant for me. Is this unusual?**

ANSWER: No, it is not unusual. Doctors sometimes use antidepressants for irritable bowel syndrome, but I do not like this approach except in the most severe cases because of the potential side effects that can accompany antidepressants.

CHAPTER 14

NATURAL SOLUTIONS FOR ARTHRITIS

Be not wise in your own eyes: reverently fear and
worship the Lord and turn [entirely] away from evil.
It shall be health to your nerves and sinews, and
marrow and moistening to your bones.
—PROVERBS 3:7–8, AMP

H URTING EVERY DAY IS NO WAY TO LIVE. In these days of modern technology, advanced medical techniques and improved hygiene, we are
living much longer than we did just a hundred years ago. Unfortunately,
many elderly people experience so much pain every day in their bodies
that they wish they could just go on to heaven. Although the major killers
are still heart disease, cancer and strokes, the number one cause of disabil-
ities is arthritis. Between rheumatoid arthritis, osteoarthritis, joint inflammation and a very painful form of arthritis called gout, it seems that we
barely have a chance to avoid it as we age. What is the point of living
eighty or ninety years on the earth if the last several decades are filled with
debilitating joint pain?

God has provided a plant and animal kingdom full of natural remedies
of which we are just becoming aware. After we become Christians, we
have a renewed spirit man, but we still have to live our lives on earth in
physical bodies. And those physical bodies need to be "renewed" just as
our spirits and minds need to be renewed.

111

Arthritis Is Not Just Affecting the Elderly

Most of us associate the degeneration of arthritis with something our grandparents had; the idea that younger people could develop arthritis may seem a bit far-fetched. In my experience, an astonishing 90 percent of all forty-year-olds have the beginning stages of cartilage degeneration. This does not mean that they are necessarily in pain or are facing disability at that point, but it does mean that without certain changes in their diet and lifestyle, there is a good chance that full-blown arthritis will develop—and not just later in life. Nearly three out of five people with arthritis are under the age of sixty-five![1]

What could be the cause of such a trend? First of all, the poor diet that most Americans consume does not contain the nutrition needed to foster healthy cartilage replacement in the joints. Not only that, but the typical diet promotes obesity in our society. And if a person is twenty pounds overweight, this weight-bearing problem is almost certainly causing arthritic changes in their joints, especially the knees and the hips.

Another reason for the growing prominence of arthritis in the younger generation is the increasing number of athletic injuries that occur. If a person has suffered a football injury, a hockey injury, a skating injury and so on, the risk of arthritis increases threefold due to the damage sustained to the cartilage in the joints.

With such alarming risks and such pain and debilitation at stake, thank God that He has made it possible to prevent and even correct the joint pain and worn-out cartilage that causes arthritis. In these days, it is becoming increasingly important to take advantage of the preventive measures that God has put in place for us. While Satan would love to keep so many of God's people bound up with the excruciating pain and joint stiffness that arthritis causes, God offers you a better plan.

Below are questions designed to determine if you are exhibiting the signs of arthritis. Answer them as accurately as you can.

1. During the past twelve months, have you had pain, aching, stiffness or swelling in or around a joint?

2. In a typical month, were these symptoms present daily for at least half of the days in the month?

3. Do you have pain in your knee or hip when climbing stairs or walking two to three blocks (¼ mile) on flat ground?

4. Do you have daily pain or stiffness in your hand joints?

5. Are you now limited in any way in any activities because of joint symptoms (pain, aching, stiffness or loss of motion)?

Your Score: If you answered *yes* to any of the questions, you are exhibiting symptoms that may be arthritis or another condition that needs to be diagnosed. You should confirm this diagnosis with your healthcare provider.

Natural Cartilage Repair

Since the underlying problem of arthritis involves the disintegration of the cartilage in the joints, the search for symptom relief as well as an ultimate cure involves focusing on three aspects of the cartilage problem:

1. Relief from the pain the destroyed cartilage has caused
2. Control of the inflammation in the joints
3. Regeneration and restoration of the destroyed cartilage

Traditional medicine has made great strides in the first two areas of focus. The first treatment for someone suffering with arthritis is to get their pain under control, and the medical community has devised numerous treatments that give patients effective pain relief. Unfortunately, many medical treatments stop at that point.

Traditional medicine's current "breakthroughs" have been taking place in the treatment of the second focus we listed: controlling the inflammation of the joints. You may have seen the deluge of commercial advertisements for medications such as Celebrex or Vioxx. Older anti-inflammatory drugs, including Advil and Aleve, were effective in shrinking the swelling in the joints, but their side effects caused multiple stomach problems, sometimes as severe as ulcers.

So scientists went to work and developed a new class of drugs that could counter inflammation effectively without the harmful side effects to the stomach. However, it is still not possible to take such a potent drug as Celebrex or Vioxx without some side effects. Rather than causing simple stomach ulcers, they interact with the kidneys, which can create serious problems for the patient.

The third focus we mentioned—rebuilding the disintegrated cartilage—has not begun to be addressed by the medical community. However, rather than deal with an array of side effects from traditional prescriptions for managing pain and inflammation of arthritis, which can be as bad, or worse, than the original problem, many people are exploring the possibility of nutritional supplements for help.

Nutritional Answers for Arthritis and Joint Problems

The wonderful news is that God has provided elements in nature to help correct these painful arthritic conditions. Some of these nutritional answers provide more than just relief from the symptoms of arthritis; they can actually *reverse* cartilage damage, restoring health to damaged cartilage caused by the disease—the aspect that traditional medicine has not even addressed.

So what should you do to cope with arthritis if you are suffering from its pain and debilitation? First of all, you should begin to seek God for His pathway to healing for *you*. Consider that your pathway could include the nutrients that God has placed in the plant and animal kingdoms, which have been there since the beginning of time. I encourage you to become acquainted with the following natural resources God has provided that have proven helpful in the treatment of this painful disease.

Curcuma

Curcuma is a substance that comes from turmeric, a plant root commonly found in curry powder. Throughout thousands of years of history, especially in the Near and Far East, people used curcuma to control the pain and swelling in their joints, even though they had no idea what its chemical structure or true medicinal value was. I have found that the newer arthritic drugs called Celebrex and Vioxx, which reduce joint inflammation, contain the same active ingredient that is present in curcuma! But better still, curcuma does not create the same kidney problems that these other medications do. I recommend 100 milligrams daily.

Tart cherries

The kind of cherries that create benefits for the joints and cartilage are not Bing cherries or the cherries you would find on top of an ice cream sundae. You would find these beneficial cherries in a cherry pie. They are the tart cherries that most people don't want to eat by themselves because they are so bitter. It is the beneficial chemical in them that causes the undesired tartness. Just as the case was with curcuma, tart cherries have been used for centuries to alleviate arthritic pain and joint swelling.

Researchers at Michigan State conducted a study on these tart cherries and found that the active ingredient used by ancient peoples for thousands of years to relieve their symptoms of arthritis was again *the same ingredient found in the prescription medications Celebrex and Vioxx.* And again, the tart cherries had none of the negative side effects that the prescription drugs did.[2] For these reasons, I recommend 100 milligrams a day of tart cherry fruit powder.

Holy basil

Holy basil is another ingredient that contains much the same properties as curcuma and tart cherries; again, it has been used for hundreds of years to bring relief to painful, swollen joints. One hundred fifty milligrams a day is sufficient to help relieve pain and reduce inflammation.

Boswellia (frankincense)

In biblical times, frankincense was a prized possession, so much so that it was among the gifts presented by the Magi—among such other costly gifts as gold and myrrh—to the very young King Jesus (Matt. 2:11). At that time, it was valued primarily for its fragrant aroma, but as people rubbed it on their joints as a perfumed ointment, they began to discover that it had healing properties as well.

Today, what was then known as frankincense is called by its chemical name of boswellia. Boswellia comes from a plant that contains the active chemical boswellic acid, now proven to be a potent anti-inflammatory substance. Initially, the gum resin of the plant was used in Bible days to spread topically on the joints, but today we have discovered that its effectiveness increases when it is taken internally.

In one study conducted on boswellia, out of one hundred fifty people given the chemical, 70 percent found that the morning stiffness in their joints disappeared altogether, and a whopping 97 percent noticed a significant improvement in their symptoms.[3] If you are suffering from arthritis, you understand that mornings are often the worst time of day for joint stiffness; as the day begins and you start to move around, the joint stiffness decreases. Boswellia, the frankincense that was presented to our King Jesus, has been shown to cause that morning stiffness to virtually disappear!

How is it able to work so effectively? The researchers found that, again, the same chemical present in the new medications Celebrex and Vioxx are active in boswellia, only, again, *without the side effects!*[4] Two hundred milligrams a day is recommended.

Sea cucumber

A sea cucumber is not a member of the plant kingdom but a marine animal, an underwater creature that feeds on plankton in every sea on earth. As the sea cucumbers, also known as bechedemer, strain the plankton, they collect certain compounds from these tiny marine organisms that have amazing anti-inflammatory properties.

Glucosamine and chondroitin

In recent years in the United States, doctors have begun to connect with the "nutritional world" in recognizing the healing properties of *glucosamine* and *chondroitin,* especially in the treatment of arthritis. Now the scientific community has been able to witness cases of arthritis where the disease is *actually reversed.*

One study recorded in the medical journal *Lancet* looked at 212 people who suffered from arthritis. Half of them were given glucosamine, and half were given a placebo. The study followed the patients for three years, and the results were amazing. Glucosamine patients showed at least a 25 percent rate of improvement in their symptoms, while the patients on the placebo got worse! Patients receiving glucosamine ultimately lost 80 percent less cartilage than their counterparts![5] What that means is that the disease was stopped, and even partially reversed, in patients who took 1,500 milligrams of glucosamine a day.

For years, doctors considered arthritis a progressive disease, meaning that once a person had it, they knew that their joints and cartilage were on a decline that would continue until their lives ended. With the use of glucosamine, however, it is possible to provide patients with a real solution. Glucosamine can *stop* the debilitating progression of the disease!

It works especially well when combined with *chondroitin,* a compound found in animal cartilage. When people take glucosamine without combining it with chondroitin, it can take the glucosamine up to three months longer to "kick in." But when the glucosamine and chondroitin are combined (along with the other natural substances that we discussed), relief can begin to occur within a matter of days. The symptoms will be quickly reduced, and over the long run, the disease can be stopped and eventually reversed.

Joint cartilage is a fascinating part of the body. Did you realize that it contains no blood vessels whatsoever? All of its nourishment comes from the fluid surrounding the joint, known as the *synovial fluid.* Each time you take a step, you are literally walking on water, because the cartilage that is surrounded by the synovial fluid is actually 90 percent water. When the cartilage wears down and the synovial fluid is depleted, the painful situation occurs in which bone rubs against bone in the joint—especially in the knee and the hip.

To repair this damage, glucosamine works to rebuild the cartilage itself, and chondroitin serves to attract the necessary water to return to the cartilage, inflating like a sponge and building the cushion back up within the joint. Glucosamine should be taken at a dose of 1,500 milligrams a day, and chondroitin at a dose of 100 milligrams a day. Additionally, sea cucumber may be taken at a dose of 100 milligrams per day.

Our God is an amazing God, full of grace and compassion for all of our needs. He has provided a way, within His natural plant and animal kingdoms, for us not only to deal with the symptoms of joint disease, but also to know how to repair the damage that was done and restore the joints to the way He intended for them to work. God is in the restoration business!

Bromelain

In the Pacific Islands, there is a much lower incidence of joint problems than there is in our own country. That fact may be attributed to their consumption of pineapple. Within the stocky portion of the pineapple, the part that most of us choose not to eat, lies a compound called *bromelain*. It too acts as an anti-inflammatory, decreasing the production of the chemicals in the body that cause swelling. One study showed that bromelain decreased inflammation in up to 60 percent of seven hundred patients who took it in its extract form. And a significant number also reported a dramatic decrease in their pain.[6] An additional study looked at 146 boxers, and those boxers who took the bromelain rather than the placebo healed from their bruises and joint injuries three times faster.

Bromelain has other healing properties as well. It can decrease blood clotting and reduce blood pressure, probably because it works as an anti-inflammatory on the arterial walls. For this reason, it is beneficial to patients with cardiovascular disease as well as to those with arthritis. Fifty milligrams a day is a sufficient dosage.

Diet and Arthritis

Traditionally, doctors have been trained to believe that a person's diet does not affect the progression or severity of arthritic symptoms. That belief is changing. Now, as the medical community is beginning to accept the validity of nutrition's impact on disease and the value of supplementation, we are learning what effect certain nutrients have on disease. For example, the omega fatty acids, specifically the omega-3s, the omega-6s and the omega-9s, have a direct effect on joint pain and swelling. In fact, if they are taken in the correct balance, these vital nutrients can even reverse the progression of arthritis.

The question has been asked, Can corn oil worsen arthritis? Surprisingly, the answer is *yes*. It is a bit ironic that several years ago, the American Heart Association recommended that the population change from cooking in saturated fats to cooking with polyunsaturated oils, such as corn oil, safflower oil, flaxseed oil and peanut oil, to protect the heart. However, these are all omega-6 fatty acids, which contain a compound called linoleic acid. In the human body, linoleic acid is converted into arachidonic acid, which is actually an inflammatory compound—that is, it causes inflammation throughout the body, including in the joints, furthering problems with arthritis and joint swelling and pain.

When the corn oils are *balanced* with the omega-3 fatty acids, found in fatty fish, the inflammation caused by omega-6 fatty acids is eliminated. Unfortunately, in the typical American diet, instead of the correct balance of a one-to-one ratio of omega-6 and omega-3 fatty acids, we have a twenty-to-one ratio! What can be done? First, begin to cut down on your use of corn oil, peanut oil and flaxseed oil, and second, increase the omega-3s in your diet, either through eating fatty fish or through a dietary supplement.

In conclusion, there are three aspects to the battle against arthritis and joint disease:

1. Reduce the pain.
2. Reduce the inflammation.
3. Stop and then reverse the cartilage damage.

Although modern medicine cannot offer viable solutions to all three of these aspects, God, in His grace, has made all things possible to you through your diligent commitment to seek His pathway for your healing. Choosing to use the substances He created in the plant and animal kingdoms for your use, you can create a battle plan against this disease. You don't have to suffer in pain anymore—begin to take the necessary steps to cure your arthritis and repair your cartilage and joints today!

🍒 ASK DR. CHERRY

QUESTION: **Is it true that exercise can strengthen the joints and help alleviate the symptoms of arthritis?**

ANSWER: Yes. The action of exercise increases the influx of water into the cartilage, increasing the cushioning. Long-distance runners have less, not more, arthritis problems.

QUESTION: **Since glucosamine comes from shellfish, which is one of God's forbidden foods listed in Leviticus 11 and Deuteronomy 14, why do you recommend it as a treatment for arthritis?**

ANSWER: The beneficial aspects of the shellfish—the part that helps restore cartilage in the joints—comes from the chitin, a part of the shellfish that actually is derived from the shell, not the meat, of the shellfish. Levitical laws refer to the *meat* of the shellfish when they forbid its consumption, and eating the meat is generally what causes health problems in people. The reason for that is because shellfish have poor filtration systems, and therefore they can accumulate high levels of bacteria within their flesh. Toxic levels of mercury and lead within the meat of shellfish have also been known to cause cholera epidemics.

God has used various unclean animals in the Bible to help people. One example is when the prophet Elijah was fed by a raven, an unclean, scavenger bird. God often works in mysterious ways through means we don't understand. You should not fear that you are violating God's law by taking glucosamine chondroitin; because it is derived from the shell, it is not forbidden.

ESSENTIAL NUTRITION FOR CARTILAGE AND JOINT FUNCTION

NUTRIENT	EFFECT	DAILY DOSAGE
Glucosamine	Nutrient that has been shown in clinical studies to reduce pain and help repair damaged cartilage[8]	1,500 mg
Chondroitin sulfate	Nutrient that works with glucosamine to protect and regenerate joint tissue	100 mg
Holy basil leaf extract	Herb that helps relieve pain and reduce inflammation by inhibiting the COX-2 enzyme	150 mg
Turmeric root powder (curcuma)	Herb that helps relieve pain and reduce inflammation by inhibiting the COX-2 enzyme	100 mg
Tart cherry fruit powder	Herb that helps relieve pain and reduce inflammation by inhibiting the COX-2 enzyme	100 mg
Boswellia serrata sap extract	Herb that has been shown to effectively reduce the discomfort of swollen joints and morning stiffness, as well as improve grip strength and physical performance	200 mg
Sea cucumber	Natural substance that acts as an anti-inflammatory agent	100 mg
Bromelain	Natural compound that reduces inflammation	50 mg

CHAPTER 15

ALZHEIMER'S DISEASE & OTHER MEMORY PROBLEMS

Then your light shall break forth like the morning,
your healing shall spring forth speedily.
—ISAIAH 58:8, NKJV

HAVE YOU EVER FORGOTTEN SOMEONE'S NAME? LOST YOUR CAR KEYS? All of us show signs of forgetfulness from time to time, especially as we get older, so where is the line drawn between simple forgetfulness and a symptom of a more dangerous, more frightening prospect—the prospect of Alzheimer's disease or another neurological disorder?

One humorous prescription for determining when forgetfulness has become a serious problem says, "It's not Alzheimer's when you forget where you put your car keys. It's Alzheimer's when you forget what the keys are for!"

The problem of neurological impairment—including Alzheimer's disease, dementia and severe memory loss—is on the rise. Reports suggest that in the next twenty-five years, the incidence of Alzheimer's disease will triple. Already 50 percent of the population that attains the age of eighty-five shows the signs of early Alzheimer's. But you don't have to be among the elderly to have problems in this area; almost everyone over the age of forty has some degree of age-related memory loss (ARML).[1]

Despite this seemingly bad news, it is important to keep in mind that the promises of God are still true and that He still wants to satisfy us with a long life lived in fullness on the earth. God's Word is very reassuring when it comes to the problem of decreasing memory and mental function. Consider the following promises:

> But God hath not given us the spirit of fear; but of power, and of love, and of a sound mind.
>
> —2 TIMOTHY 1:7

> For God is not the author of confusion, but of peace.
>
> —1 CORINTHIANS 14:33

Confusion may result in losing your car keys! More seriously, confusion occurs in the mind of the Alzheimer's patient who can no longer remember the names of his precious wife and children. God is saying that confusion is not His way–it's not His plan! He has made a way possible for you to walk in divine health, to maintain a sound mind all of your days.

A Doctor's Test for Alzheimer's Disease

Many people begin to forget little things here and there as they age. This forgetfulness causes them to wonder, *Do I have Alzheimer's disease? Am I going to lose my mind?* The key to determining whether or not the problem is serious is to determine whether or not it is *progressive*.

Let me give you an example. Let's consider Tom, a businessman in his early fifties. One day as he is sitting at his office desk, he looks around for his favorite fountain pen and discovers it is missing. This has happened a few times, and he wonders, *Why do I keep losing this pen?* He finds it a few minutes later, right where he had left it; the pen had simply been misplaced. Tom thinks no further of it until he begins to notice he is forgetting names of acquaintances, and then names of close friends whom he has known for years. Finally one day, to his consternation, he gets into his car and realizes he cannot remember the way home from work.

In the earlier stages of this man's forgetfulness, there was no real cause for alarm, but once it became progressive, causing him to forget more and more familiar pieces of information, a more serious problem became obvious.

To determine the cause of a possible problem, doctors use a standard memory test. They will state three words aloud to the patient—such as *run, blue, table*—and then tell the person that they will be asked to repeat those words two minutes later in the conversation. Whether or not the patient can complete this task successfully tells the doctor a great deal about the functioning of the memory centers of the patient's brain.

When the doctor states the words, they are stored as a memory and sent down to the entorhinal area of the brain, and finally to the hippocampus, where longer-term memories are stored. Because Alzheimer's affects these areas of the brain first, it is possible to pinpoint potential early Alzheimer's patients if they fail the test.

However, some degree of forgetfulness can be caused by distraction or a lack of attention at the time the information is given. The distraction prevents the listener from incorporating what was heard and moving it into the memory centers of the brain. For that reason, doctors will additionally ask the patient about memories from his or her childhood. If the patient cannot remember these memories as well, it is a strong indication that something is causing a serious impairment in the brain. Most early Alzheimer's patients would be able to recall childhood memories, but the majority of them would not be able to repeat the list of words. So doctors work backward to find out where the degree of forgetfulness begins and determine the level of impairment from there.

By the way, can you remember the three words we listed before? If you said, "Run, blue, table," you are right, and your short-term memory seems to be working just fine!

Symptoms of Serious Memory Impairment

There are certain symptoms that neurologists check for when they are considering a diagnosis of Alzheimer's or serious memory impairment. The following are the most common, which I have listed so that you can be aware of developing problems and take steps to avoid a potential crisis.

Short-term memory loss

As I mentioned previously, when doctors give patients three words to remember and then repeat a few minutes later, the majority of those who later developed Alzheimer's were unable to remember two out of the three.

Problems with simple arithmetic

Alzheimer's patients have great difficulty performing calculations or simple arithmetic in their minds. These are not calculations such as finding the square root of 302. These calculations are the simple addition and subtraction problems that we learned as children, such as two plus five equals seven.

Repetition

Now just because your old uncle Joe likes to retell his famous fishing story over and over about when he caught the biggest bass in the county, it doesn't mean that he is in the early stages of Alzheimer's. But if people repeat the same story over and over again, because they can't remember that they just told it five minutes ago, it signals a problem. If a person asks the same question over and over again, because they don't remember having asked it moments prior, there is some degree of short-term memory loss that has already developed.

Getting lost in familiar places

If a person has taken the same route home from work for ten years, but one day cannot remember which way to go, it is a warning sign; a doctor should probably be consulted.

Poor judgment

This is not the poor judgment that a young person might have when he or she makes bad decisions that are based on immaturity. When people suddenly begin to wear soiled clothing or forget to bathe, they are exercising poor judgment because of their mental state. Another example is when a woman continually forgets to turn off the oven or a man leaves the car running in the driveway because he forgot to turn the motor off.

Forgetting names

Forgetting the names of strangers or one-time acquaintances does not usually signal a significant problem. However, a person has already developed a serious problem when he or she can't remember the name of their aunt or uncle, or their closest friend for thirty years, or that of their own mother or child.

Any one of these symptoms may not be an indication of too serious of a problem, but if more than one symptom begins to manifest, and if there are signs of progressive memory loss, it's time to consider getting some help for the problem.

Natural Remedies for Memory Loss

Until just recently, the medical community has believed that once a neuron, a nerve cell, died—including the cells of the brain—it could never be regenerated, or brought back to life. They believed the body could heal itself in every other tissue or organ, but once damage was done in the brain, it was irreversible.

Within the last two to three years, scientists have begun to learn that brain cells, or neurons, can and do regenerate under the proper conditions. The following natural substances are proven remedies for improving memory function as well as stopping the progress of the devastating Alzheimer's disease.

Huperzine-A (club moss)

When the brain's nerve cells communicate among themselves, they send signals to the various parts of the body to perform their various functions—the heart to beat, the lungs to breathe, the feet to walk and so on. This critical communication occurs because of the various chemicals that move in areas between the cells, called synapses. The chemical that communicates memories between these neurons is called *acetylcholine*. As you age, the level of acetylcholine in your brain begins to decrease, and as a result, your memory function begins to deteriorate.

In modern medicine, there are a number of drugs that serve to increase the chemical acetylcholine in our brains and thus promote good memory. These include Aricept, Cognex, Exelon and Reminyl, but they are very expensive and, like all man-made drugs, have side effects.

A natural source of the chemical huperzine-A, which amazingly has been found to increase acetylcholine levels just as effectively as prescription drugs, is synthesized from the club moss plant. It does this by inhibiting the enzyme that breaks down acetylcholine in the brain, thus allowing the levels to increase. The club moss plant has increased memory, thinking ability, focus and concentration in many Alzheimer's patients. The recommended dosage is 0.1 milligrams daily.

Interestingly, the Chippewa Indian tribe, which lived on the east coast of the United States hundreds of years ago, knew to seek out the club moss plant to improve their memory—*and they sought out the very two species of this plant that increased the acetylcholine levels!* The same can be said for the Chinese culture hundreds of years ago and halfway around the globe. God loves all of His people everywhere, and He has made provision in His creation for all of the nations to be blessed!

Periwinkle (vinpocetine)

For years, periwinkle, because of a chemical found in it called vincristine, has been used in traditional treatments for cancer. But about twenty years ago, scientists began to learn that another potent chemical in periwinkle, vinpocetine, had helpful properties in dealing with memory loss. Although it is primarily used in Europe, vinpocetine is gaining popularity in the United States. Its primary function in the body is as a vasodilator, meaning that it causes the blood vessels to dilate, or open up, to a greater extent. The reason this improves memory function is that it enlarges the blood vessels to the brain, allowing more oxygen and nutrient supply to the brain.

The human brain is a very selfish organ of the body. Even though it requires only about 2 percent of the space within the body, it demands about 20 percent of the oxygen and the glucose as its primary energy source. Other cells and tissues are able to utilize either glucose or fat, but the brain does not offer this choice. It requires glucose, which must be delivered through the bloodstream.

So, when a natural substance works to cause the blood vessels to the brain to enlarge, it increases the blood supply to the brain, which is carrying its vital needs for functioning: oxygen and glucose. When these levels are raised in the brain, the person's memory and concentration will improve, and their absentmindedness and confusion will begin to disappear. One milligram daily is the recommended dose.

Phosphatidylserine (PS)

Phosphatidylserine (PS) is a phospholipid of the human body that is used as the primary building block in the lining of the nerve cell, or nerve sheath, but PS is also present in the soybean plant. When it is added as a supplement to the diet, it can improve failing memory and learning ability in people with ARML (age-related memory loss) in as little as three months!

This improvement takes place because the PS increases and strengthens the membranes of the nerve cells in the brain along which the electrical impulses of communication pass. It also helps glucose, the fuel of the brain, to be absorbed better and thus increase the energy level of the entire brain. When there is better neuron communication and greater brain energy, memory and concentration begin to improve significantly. One hundred milligrams is the recommended daily dose.

Ginkgo

Perhaps the most well-known supplement proven to increase mental function and memory is the extract that comes from the ginkgo tree. Interestingly, the ginkgo tree is the oldest surviving species of tree on earth—it even survived the detonation of the atomic bomb in Hiroshima during World War II. Within the leaves of this hardy plant comes a substance that produces amazing results.

One of the primary functions of ginkgo in the body is to dilate the blood vessels and provide a greater flow of oxygen and nutrients to the brain, much like the action of the periwinkle plant. However, because ginkgo also works as a blood thinner, patients who are already on blood thinners, such as Coumadin, should be careful to take only small amounts of ginkgo. Instead, combine it with one of these other listed nutrient remedies and allow God to bring healing to both your blood pressure and your mental functions.

For someone without blood pressure problems, the recommended dosage is 100 milligrams per day.

B vitamins

Vitamin B_{12} has had such a potent effect on preventing the effects of aging nerve cells that it has actually been called the "senility vitamin"! Vitamin B_6 is commonly known as a nerve supplement and has been used successfully in the treatment of carpal tunnel syndrome, which is essentially nerve damage in the wrist. This same nerve repair can be done in the brain through a dose of vitamin B_6. Folic acid decreases homocystine levels, but it also signals the body to produce more serotonin, a neurotransmitter that promotes communication among the nerve cells.

Vitamin B_6 should be taken at a dose of 6 milligrams per day, while vitamin B_{12} should be taken at 12 micrograms per day. The recommended dose for folic acid is 100 micrograms per day.

Vitamin E

Among people who were taking vitamin E for rheumatoid arthritis, scientists began to find less and less incidence of Alzheimer's disease or other mental difficulties. Eventually it was determined that its anti-inflammatory properties, which were so helpful in dealing with the arthritis, were also helpful in decreasing any slight inflammation within the brain that could impair its functioning. Some other natural anti-inflammatories include curry powder and tart cherries, which were discussed in chapter 14.

Each of these natural substances can make a great difference in the problem of Alzheimer's disease and memory loss, but the greatest improvements take place when all of these nutrients are allowed to work together in synergy, multiplying their effects.

We are living in a generation like no other generation—our world is full of pesticides, herbicides and pollution, all of which take a toll on our bodies—not just our lungs, blood pressure or immune systems, but on our nerve and brain cells as well. Thank God for His provision through the natural plant kingdom, which gives us a way to protect ourselves!

ASK DR. CHERRY

QUESTION: **What's all the buzz about ginkgo biloba?**

ANSWER: Ginkgo biloba, often referred to as just "ginkgo," is one of the world's most popular herbs and has been in use for some five thousand years. Derived from the world's oldest living tree species, ginkgo leaves are known to have a profound effect on brain function.

Research has shown that ginkgo increases circulation of the blood to the brain, protects brain cells from free-radical damage and enhances chemical communication between brain cells. For many people, these effects result in improved memory and an enhanced ability to focus and concentrate.

Over a dozen well-designed clinical studies have confirmed ginkgo's ability to bolster mental function. This effect has been observed in people of all ages, but it is most pronounced in those over the age of fifty.

QUESTION: **Should I take gingko if I am also taking a prescription blood thinner?**

ANSWER: Be cautious about taking supplements if you are on a prescription blood thinner, such as Coumadin. Many supplements, including gingko, can increase the effectiveness of blood thinners. Check with your doctor to see which supplements are safe for you to take. Also, get your blood levels checked regularly.

QUESTION: **The club moss that improves memory affects the neurotransmitters in the brain. I have heard that antidepressants also affect the neurotransmitters. Can the club moss improve the symptoms of depression?**

A NSWER: While it is true that both club moss and
affect the neurotransmitters in the brain, each affect
of neurotransmitters. The neurotransmitters involved in
serotonin and dopamine, but the club moss affects the neu
acetylcholine.

ESSENTIAL NUTRIENTS TO IMPROVE YOUR MIND

NUTRIENT	EFFECT	DAILY DOSAGE
Ginkgo biloba leaf extract	Herb that increases blood flow and oxygen transport to the brain and helps brain cells communicate	100 mg
Huperzine-A	Herbal extract that helps maintain healthy levels of acetylcholine, a key neurotransmitter for learning and memory	0.1 mg
Phosphatidylserine complex	Nutrient that enhances the production of neurotransmitters and helps promote memory function	100 mg
Vinpocetine	Herbal extract that improves memory function by enhancing circulation to the brain	1 mg
Vitamin B$_6$	Essential vitamin that enhances communication between brain cells and protects the brain by lowering homocysteine levels	6 mg
Vitamin B$_{12}$	Essential vitamin that improves mental function and protects brain cells by lowering homocysteine levels	12 mcg
Folic acid	Essential vitamin that promotes normal growth and development of nerve tissue and protects brain cells by lowering homocysteine levels	100 mcg

CHAPTER 16

FREEDOM FROM DEPRESSION & ANXIETY

He heals the brokenhearted and
binds up their wounds.
—PSALM 147:3, NIV

IN TODAY'S SOCIETY, DEPRESSION IS BECOMING AN INCREASINGLY COMMON PROBLEM. Depression can take the form of anxiety, sadness and eating disorders—resulting in weight loss, weight gain, sleep disturbances and numerous other problems. The common denominator to all types of depression in the physical realm is a neurotransmitter brain chemical known as *serotonin*. Literally thousands of studies have shown that adding serotonin to the body can relieve the symptoms of depression and anxious depression, and it can help patients lose weight and normalize sleep patterns.

Because it is not possible to give a person serotonin directly, the traditional medical approach has been to use a class of drugs known as SSRIs (selective serotonin reuptake inhibitors). These SSRIs prevent the reuptake of serotonin in the brain, which logically results in increased levels of serotonin. A decreased level of serotonin frequently causes depression, anxiety and other symptoms.

In general, the SSRIs are safe, and literally millions of prescriptions for them have been used. Drugs in this category include Prozac, Zoloft, Paxil, Celexa, Luvox and others. As with any drug, there are side effects in certain individuals, but generally they are well tolerated. Rarely, more serious problems occur in which patients experience unusual outbursts of temper and violence. Occasional episodes of nervousness and fatigue have also been observed.

Low serotonin levels are now implicated in a much wider variety of diseases than just depression. Some of these include sleep disorders, binge eating, attention deficit disorders, headaches, PMS, and food and carbohydrate cravings that commonly lead to obesity.

The Serotonin Solution

God created certain chemicals—amino acids—that the body naturally converts to serotonin, which can help us achieve an increase in serotonin levels. There are several chemicals in this category, but one that has aroused particular enthusiasm is an extract from a plant seed called *Griffonia Simplicifolia*. This seed contains an important chemical called 5-hydroxytryptophan (5-HTP), which helps to normalize the levels of our critical brain chemical serotonin.

The wonder of 5-HTP

Usually, the body uses an amino acid called L-tryptophan to convert to serotonin in the human body. Tryptophan occurs naturally in milk, turkey and other foods. (This is probably why you get sleepy after eating a turkey dinner or drinking a warm glass of milk at night.) Before tryptophan is converted to the beneficial brain transmitter serotonin, it is first converted to 5-HTP. However, when you ingest 5-HTP directly, as a supplement extracted from the *Griffonia* seed, 70 percent of it is converted to serotonin, compared to 3 to 5 percent of the tryptophan from the foods you eat.

I have found that 5-HTP not only helps with depression but also with anxiety symptoms. Many patients do not realize that anxiety can be part of true depression, although this seems like somewhat of a paradox. Another benefit is that these neurotransmitter chemicals in the brain can have a direct effect on appetite, and 5-HTP can help overweight patients achieve weight loss. Insomnia, which is also common with depression, also decreases markedly when the patient is on this natural supplement.

5-HTP will often produce results when traditional prescription antidepressants fail. One study involved ninety-nine patients whose conditions did not respond to any attempts at alleviating their depression. They were given the supplement 5-HTP at dosages averaging 200 milligrams daily and ranging as high as 600 milligrams daily. Nearly half of these patients had a complete recovery![1] It would certainly make sense that if 5-HTP works so well in these hard-to-treat patients, it would work even better in the more commonly encountered mild to moderate depression.

In my clinical experience, I have found that 5-HTP was equal to or better than the typically prescribed antidepressants. A major advantage was that it not only worked, but also the side effects typically were very mild, with the most frequent being mild nausea occurring in less than 10 percent of all patients. However, because 5-HTP is eliminated through the kidneys, patients with renal disease should avoid 5-HTP, as should those patients with peptic ulcer disease.

There are many other neurotransmitters in the brain that are critically important, including dopamine and norepinephrine. Serotonin appears to be one of the most prominent, and amazingly we now have a God-created chemical that can have a direct effect on the increasingly common problem of depression.

For mild to moderate depression, a dose of 50 milligrams of 5-HTP three times daily for two weeks is a good starting point. The dosage can be increased to 100 milligrams three times daily if improvement is not seen. Coated capsules or tablets are now available, which seem to decrease the nausea that patients might experience.

Weight loss

It has been noted for some time that prescription antidepressants that increase serotonin levels can help certain patients lose weight. Since 5-HTP directly increases serotonin levels, it comes as no surprise that it could function as a weight-loss aid.

Though causes for weight gain and obesity are complex, they may be related, in part, to a decreased conversion of the common amino acid tryptophan to 5-HTP, which results in lowered serotonin levels. In my experience, supplements of 5-HTP were able to reduce high-caloric intake, resulting in weight loss even though the patients made no conscious effort to lose weight.

5-HTP also produced a feeling of satiety (the feeling of satisfaction), which results from normalizing serotonin levels. Patients who were on the 5-HTP supplements tended to get full more quickly and simply were not as hungry. I would recommend starting out at a dose of perhaps 50 to 100 milligrams three times daily, and then increasing the dosage gradually.

Headache relief

Many types of recurrent chronic headaches are now associated with serotonin imbalances. This knowledge has produced a new generation of prescription medications that affect serotonin receptors, such as Imitrex and Maxalt. Because of the effect of 5-HTP on serotonin, there have been several clinical studies performed on headaches, including both tension-type headaches and migraine headaches, and the results have been excellent.[2]

Stopping insomnia

Several studies have shown the beneficial effects of 5-HTP in correcting sleep disorders. It is common knowledge that low serotonin levels can lead to chronic sleep disorders. 5-HTP has helped promote sleep by causing patients to go to sleep more quickly and stay asleep longer. I recommend a dosage of 100 to 300 milligrams forty-five minutes before going to bed at night. It is wiser to start with the lower dose and gradually increase it after about three days.

Weight gain, headaches and insomnia can indirectly cause depression in and of themselves. 5-HTP provides relief from these problems as well as improving the depression itself; therefore, it is very effective in fighting depression and anxiety.

ASK DR. CHERRY

QUESTION: **Does St. John's wort help at all to alleviate depression?**

ANSWER: Yes, it is helpful in mild to moderate cases of depression. Recent studies have shown, however, that it is not strong enough to deal with cases of severe depression.

QUESTION: **Do serotonin levels in the brain have any effect at all on fibromyalgia symptoms?**

ANSWER: Serotonin levels are low in people who have fibromyalgia and other pain disorders. Prescription medications are widely used to treat these disorders, but 5-HTP is proving to be an extremely useful supplement with fibromyalgia, which is characterized by multiple tender points throughout the body. 5-HTP is helpful in counteracting the chronic pain, fatigue and depression that accompany fibromyalgia. Dosages for fibromyalgia patients should begin at 50 milligrams three times daily and increase to 100 milligrams three times daily after two to three weeks, if adequate responses are not noted.

CHAPTER 17

TREATING HEADACHES & DIZZINESS

Bless the LORD, O my soul: and all that is within
me, bless his holy name. Bless the LORD, O my
soul, and forget not all his benefits: Who forgiveth
all thine iniquities; who healeth all thy diseases.
—PSALM 103:1–3

HEADACHES AND DIZZINESS ARE AMONG THE MOST COMMON AIL-MENTS. Fortunately, God is in the healing business, and He has provided natural treatments within His world to bring relief from these debilitating problems. Headaches are classified according to symptoms and cause. The vast majority of headaches can be relieved with simple relaxation techniques and by avoiding any unusual stimulation. Avoiding light and noise, relaxing in a quiet environment and even praying can often relieve the pain of headaches.

Types of Headaches

Categories of headaches range from simple stress or tension headaches to more severe problems such as brain tumors or temporal arteritis, which can be serious. The simple headache consists of a buzzing or pulsing discomfort in the head, and it can be related to high blood pressure, fever,

135

stress, weather and other causes. The following list may help you identify the type of headache(s) you experience.

Ice pick headaches

These are brief stabbing headaches, which, although potentially frightening to many patients, are benign.

Tension headaches

This very common headache usually begins in the back of the head or neck area, or in the forehead or temple region, and spreads throughout the head. Frequently, tension headaches occur on both sides of the head.

Cluster headaches

This type of headache is characterized by a piercing or burning pain, often occurring on one side of the head, usually in exactly the same place from one episode to another. These headaches occur on a regular basis for days or weeks at a time and then may disappear.

Migraine headaches

Migraine headaches are often referred to as "sick" headaches because vomiting, nausea and vision problems often accompany them. These headaches are due to constrictions and dilations in blood vessels in the brain. Migraines are sometimes very difficult to diagnose as they may present only with blurred vision or partial loss of a vision field on one side.

Ocular migraine headache

This type of headache can cause a loss of peripheral vision. It is often hereditary.

Combination headache

The combination headache presents as a migraine headache followed by a dull, continuing pain afterward.

Natural Pain Relief

Herbal treatments have been utilized to treat headaches. The natural, non-addictive tranquilizer kava kava can help to relieve tension headaches. A migraine headache, however, which is caused by the expansion and constriction of blood vessels, is better treated with feverfew and ginkgo biloba. (Simply follow the instructions on the bottle for the appropriate dosage.)

Another treatment is to add just a few drops (four to five) of fresh lemon to a cup of black coffee and then sip it slowly. Caffeine is a well-known, plant-derived substance that can help alleviate headaches by dilating the blood vessels in the brain. Another herbal treatment is to apply cold compresses that have had two to three drops of peppermint oil added to the cloth. Placing this against the painful area for fifteen minutes can relieve simple tension headaches.

A tried-and-true remedy used by many people is to make a compress of grated horseradish added to a small amount of water and applied to a cloth. The cloth is then applied to the neck area for up to five minutes. This compress can help to extinguish the tension type of headache pain.

Try not to get into the habit of using large amounts of caffeine-containing, over-the-counter compounds on a regular basis. This can lead to the phenomenon known as "rebound headaches." This simply means that as the caffeine levels decrease in your bloodstream, the headache will return, and you will require more and more caffeine-containing medication to stop it. If all other methods fail, there are some newer prescription-type medications available, such as Maxalt and Zomig, which may provide relief.

Dizziness

Dizziness is one of the most common neurological symptoms encountered in the medical practice. It is, in fact, second only to fatigue among "non-pain" symptoms. On one end of the scale, dizziness is often a vague complaint that can be very brief and benign. By the same token, it can extend to more serious diseases such as tumors or decreased blood flow to the brain.

The most common form of dizziness is known as *vertigo*. This term describes a sensation of motion when there is no motion or an exaggerated sense of motion in response to certain body movements. Vertigo may be a "spinning sensation," but it can also be a sense of falling forward, falling backward or tumbling. Most forms of vertigo are related to inner ear problems, often accompanied by nausea, vomiting and occasional hearing loss.

The inner ear serves as a primary balance mechanism that involves canals lined with small hairlike structures. Within the canals are tiny crystals made of calcium carbonate, which press against the small hairs. These small crystals, known as *otoliths*, move as our body position changes, and gravity causes the crystals to press against hairs in different positions and send signals to the brain that orient us and keep us steady.

To maintain our balance, God created a complex series of organs that interact with each other. These include the inner ear, muscles, eyes and even pressure receptors in the skin. All of these organs provide input to the brain. The brain processes these signals to keep us in a steady balance.

Poor circulation to the brain can cause dizziness, as can certain viral or bacterial infections. Abnormally high or low blood pressure and brain tumors are also causes of dizziness. Anemia can result in dizziness as well, due to an inadequate oxygen supply to various organs.

Many patients become unnecessarily distraught due to a sudden onset of vertigo in the form of spinning or dizziness. However, although it can be extremely upsetting, in most cases it is benign and can be treated with simple measures. In fact, one of the most common forms of vertigo is called "benign positional vertigo." This is a spinning sensation that is associated with changes in head position, particularly when the person is lying down and suddenly sits up or stands. This form of vertigo tends to be brief and episodic, whereas viral or bacterial infections can cause an almost constant vertigo for several days and then disappear as the body's immune system functions take over.

When we suddenly rise from a sitting or stooped over position and feel dizzy for a few seconds, it is caused by a temporary drop in blood pressure, known as *orthostatic hypotension.* If this occurs, it is almost always harmless, unless it occurs frequently. If that is the case, it could be indicating that the person has a consistently low blood pressure.

To be certain there is not a more serious problem, a physician should evaluate any kind of persistent vertigo or dizziness. Occasionally an MRI is ordered to rule out any more dangerous conditions.

Natural Relief for Dizziness

God has provided several natural nutrients that can bring relief from the common problem of dizziness.

B vitamins

All of the B vitamins are important for normal brain and nervous system function. Taking a complex of the water-soluble B vitamins as part of your daily nutrient supplements is critical in maintaining a healthy nervous system. One hundred milligrams of vitamin B_3 taken three times daily can be very useful because of its effect on cerebral circulation. However, this dosage should not be taken if you have high blood pressure or liver problems.

Extra B complex, 100 milligrams two to three times daily, as well as extra B_6, 50 milligrams daily, may be helpful during periods of dizziness. Up to 1,000 micrograms of vitamin B_{12} daily can also be useful.

Other supplements

I recommend vitamin C, 2,000 milligrams daily, and vitamin E, 800 IU (natural form) daily, for dizziness. Coenzyme Q_{10}, when taken at a dose of 90 to 150 milligrams daily, can be useful during periods of dizziness as well.

Ginger

Certain herbs, such as powdered whole gingerroot in doses of 500 to 1,000 milligrams, can relieve dizziness and nausea. Ginger has been consumed for thousands of years to help treat dizziness. In one study of sailors who consumed 1 gram of powdered ginger two to three times daily, there were markedly reduced symptoms associated with seasickness, such as vomiting and dizziness.[1] Ginger is available in capsules and can be taken thirty minutes before dizziness is anticipated and then every one to two hours thereafter.

Ginkgo

Ginkgo extract has been used for the treatment of vertigo in European countries. A typical dose should be 40 milligrams three times daily. Ginkgo extract can also improve blood circulation to the brain, as we have discussed.

Remember God's promise! If you diligently hearken to His voice, He will allow none of the diseases that affect the rest of the world to afflict you. (See Exodus 15:26.) As you develop an understanding of how headaches and dizziness attack your body, you will be better able to pray effectively and stand against them.

If you are experiencing a problem with headaches, sudden vertigo or dizziness, you should pray about your specific pathway to healing. Let the Holy Spirit guide you and give you wisdom. Consider utilizing these natural treatments from God's plant kingdom. His desire is that you experience perfect health in your body and freedom from pain and dizzy spells.

ASK DR. CHERRY

QUESTION: **At what point should I see my doctor about my frequent headaches? Can migraine headaches indicate a brain tumor?**

ANSWER: Three or more severe headaches or a sudden onset of a different type of headache signal the need to see a doctor. Fortunately, true migraine headaches have no connection to brain tumors.

QUESTION: **Why does dizziness seem to occur more frequently in older people?**

ANSWER: As I discussed before, the small crystals within the ear canals, known as otoliths, help us sense our gravitational position and maintain our balance. However, as we get older, small amounts of debris can accumulate in the canals of the inner ear and activate the hair cells, resulting in false signals.

CHAPTER 18

REMEDIES FOR VISION PROBLEMS

Moses was 120 years old when he died,
yet his eyesight was perfect and he was
as strong as a young man.
—DEUTERONOMY 34:7, TLB

W E NEVER LOSE OUR WONDER OF *ENJOYING THE VIEW!* Of all the senses in the human body, people cherish their vision more than any other. God understands this, and He has much to say in His Word about our eyesight. The writer of Proverbs instructs us clearly in this regard:

Listen, son of mine, to what I say. Listen carefully. Keep these thoughts ever in mind; let them penetrate deep within your heart, for they will mean real life for you and radiant health...Look straight ahead; don't even turn your head to look. Watch your step. Stick to the path and be safe.
—PROVERBS 4:20–22, 25–26, TLB

First of all, we are to pay attention to God's Word in order to receive the life and radiant health that God wants us to experience. But to do that, we are to look straight ahead of us to follow the path that He wants us to go. We need our eyesight to see His path! We especially need it to be able to study His Word, to keep it before our eyes so that the path remains clear.

The biblical record of Moses' death tells us something unusual about his health. It records for us the fact that Moses was 120 years old when he died and that his "eye was not dim, nor his natural force abated" (Deut. 34:7). The Living Bible paraphrase of this verse says, "His eyesight was perfect and he was as strong as a young man." Even in old age, Moses did not experience cataracts, macular degeneration or other vision problems that most of us experience as we get older. Thank God that we don't have to be like everybody else! He has a better way for His children.

Where should you turn when you begin to experience problems with your vision, those early symptoms that indicate something is going wrong, or worse, a full-blown diagnosis that could indicate encroaching blindness? Psalm 121 gives us the answer:

> *I will lift up mine eyes unto the hills, from whence cometh my help. My help cometh from the LORD, which made heaven and earth.*
>
> —PSALM 121:1–2

God is our source of healing, and He is interested in curing both our spiritual and our physical blindness. He Himself is light, and He longs to dispel all darkness from our lives. Begin to seek Him for the pathway He would have you take to protect your precious eyesight. If you are already experiencing vision problems, ask Him to show you the pathway to healing He has prepared for you.

Common Vision Problems

Do you wear glasses or have eye problems? Are you concerned your vision isn't as sharp as it used to be? Your eyes are a delicate and sensitive part of your body, and aging, pollution and sun exposure can weaken or damage them.

The primary vision problems that people have as they age include cataracts, macular degeneration, glaucoma and retinopathy—the damage caused to the blood vessels of the eyes that is often related to diabetes. Let's take a look at each of these—what is occurring within the eye and the natural substances God has placed in our world that can stop or even reverse the process of these diseases.

Cataracts

Worldwide, the greatest cause of blindness is cataracts. In the United States, there are surgical procedures that can stop blindness before it occurs, but when you consider that other countries don't have our technology, it's easy to see how cataracts can become such a problem.

Still, even here in our country, when the doctor gives someone a diagnosis of cataracts, he generally sends the patient home "to see what develops." Well, usually what happens is the cataract gets worse, until surgery becomes required to save the person's vision. Thousands of cataract surgeries are performed every year in this country—in fact, it is the most performed surgery in the United States, even above appendectomies and gallbladder surgery. Over four billion dollars are spent on cataract surgery every year in this country. Wouldn't it be so much better to find a simpler way to stop the progress of cataracts at the very beginning stages?

Early signs that you are developing cataracts is that you begin to notice fogginess in your vision, a film over your eyes. Often, while driving at night, the streetlights will begin to bother you because the way the light hits the cataract causes you to see what looks like halos around the lights. What is occurring is a degradation of the proteins within the lens of the eye, which causes a distortion in the person's vision.

Someone has said that if you live long enough, you are certain to develop cataracts. We, as Christians, don't accept that as truth, because God has provided us with ways to counter the progressive damage to the eyes that occurs as we grow older.

Macular degeneration

The leading cause of irreversible blindness in the United States, not worldwide as we discussed with the problem of cataracts, is macular degeneration. Many older Americans, especially as they continue to age, have age-related macular degeneration. What causes this problem, and more importantly, what can be done about it?

The *macula* is a small area in the back of the eye, in the retina where the central focus of light takes place. When eye doctors observe the macula in the retina, it appears as a small, concentrated yellow spot. Light passes into the eye through the lens and is magnified and focused down onto the retina, more specifically onto the macula where the sharpest focus of vision takes place.

Sunlight can be very harmful to the little macula. Within the prism of sunlight, the most dangerous rays are blue in color. If too many blue rays are allowed to come into contact with the macula, it destroys the nerve endings, and the person's vision will eventually begin to break down, causing *macular degeneration.*

Because macular degeneration can creep up on a person very slowly, it is important to pay attention to any early warning signs that may develop. One of the first symptoms is the loss of the central vision. A person begins to have trouble reading, doing close-up work, driving, seeing colors or even distinguishing faces. The big tip-off is that people with macular degeneration can see things on the side of their vision much more clearly than right in the center. One of the first things people notice is that when they walk through a doorway, and they are trying to focus on the center of the door, the frames begin to seem wavy as they walk through the door—this is a classic early sign of macular degeneration.

Sadly, traditional medicine has no answer for macular degeneration. The vast majority of the cases diagnosed by medical doctors are untreatable by the world's standards. Thank God that He is concerned about our eyesight, enough so that He has already put the necessary plants and natural substances in place to bring His light back into our eyes. As we will see, it is possible to completely halt the progress of macular degeneration by following God's dietary plan.

Diabetic retinopathy

As we discussed in the chapter on diabetes, this disease wreaks havoc on various areas of the body because of the negative effect it has on blood vessels that support so many different body organs. Diabetics are at a much greater risk of going blind than the general population because of the damage diabetes causes to the blood vessels of the retina.

Glaucoma

Glaucoma is a problem that occurs as pressure, for various reasons, increases in the eye. It is a relatively common cause of blindness as the pressure in the eye exerts pressure on the optic nerve. Again, there is not much medical doctors can do to treat this condition, except to prescribe eye drops to try to lower the pressure and prevent blindness from taking place. The good news is that God has provided natural substances within His world that can make a greater difference, with less cost and side effects to endure than conventional medications!

Natural Remedies for Vision Problems

Many of the natural substances help more than one type of vision problem. We will discuss the following substances that God has provided for us to maintain our good vision and correct any eye diseases or vision problems that might develop.

Lutein and zeaxanthin

The plant products *lutein* and *zeaxanthin* (types of yellow pigmentation) are found in various types of greens, such as kale, collard greens, spinach and to a lesser degree in romaine lettuce, broccoli, zucchini, squash, green peas, brussels sprouts and sweet corn.

These substances work to help prevent or stop the progress of macular degeneration by enhancing the yellow pigmentation of the macula, the pigmentation that is lost upon exposure to the sunlight. It literally functions as a sunscreen, blocking these most dangerous rays, the blue rays of the prism. Unfortunately, as our diets have worsened throughout the last several decades, most Americans do not consume enough kale and spinach to support the lutein levels that are needed to maintain good eyesight. Our poor diets have had a direct effect on the number of cases of macular degeneration that are now being reported. This is an example of how many people, because they have ignored God's dietary laws, have made themselves vulnerable to the most common cause of irreversible blindness.

But let's consider how easy it is to prevent. Every time you eat a big plate of spinach, you are literally putting a pair of heavy-duty sunglasses on the back of your eyes and protecting your eyesight from any potential damage from the sun! Fortunately, since the thought of kale and spinach doesn't appeal to many of us, you can also take lutein and zeaxanthin in supplement form. I recommend 6 milligrams per day.

These two nutrients are very helpful in preventing macular degeneration among most people, but it is especially important for those people who have the greatest risk of developing the disease. These people would include those who work or spend a great deal of time outside, being exposed to the sun's rays, or those who have blue or light-colored eyes, which are not able to filter out the harmful rays of the sun. If you have already been diagnosed with macular degeneration, take heart. Studies have shown that the pigments that have been lost can actually be restored through supplementation with lutein and zeaxanthin. In fact, within forty days of beginning a lutein supplement, studies have shown up to a 40 percent increase in the amount of protective yellow pigment present in the macula.[1]

Bilberry

In World War II, Royal Air Force pilots from Great Britain began noticing that when they ate bilberry jam and toast just before a night flight, there was a significant improvement in their night vision as they flew their fighter planes over enemy territory. The curiosity of scientists was aroused, and they began experiments to see if bilberry jam actually improved eyesight. In fact, they discovered that bilberry—a cousin of the blueberry—causes significant improvement in patients with macular degeneration.

Bilberry is also helpful for retinopathy, the damage done by diabetes to the retinal blood vessels, as well as for cataracts. When most doctors diagnose cataracts, they generally send the patient home until the problem escalates to the point where surgery is necessary. But if, at that time, the patient begins a regimen of bilberry, the progression of the cataract can be halted in its tracks. A dose of 40 milligrams per day is sufficient.

Eyebright

Eyebright comes from the Euphrasia plant, which grows wild throughout Europe. For centuries it has been used on that continent to relieve minor eye problems, especially those that deal with irritation, such as watery eyes caused by allergies, hay fever or conjunctivitis. Although eyebright does not actually counter some of the more major diseases of the eye, it does help to alleviate some of the worst symptoms associated with these diseases. I recommend 10 milligrams of eyebright daily.

Glutathione

Glutathione is already naturally present in the eyes, more concentrated in the lens. It is beneficial because it is a strong antioxidant that can counter the negative effects of free-radical formation caused by the high levels of light and oxygen that enter the eye through the lens. These free radicals are what degrade the proteins in the lens, causing cataracts to form. So, if glutathione is present in the lens, it helps in the prevention of cataracts.

Higher levels of glutathione can be found in such foods as almonds, walnuts and avocados. When used in combination with alpha lipoic acid, glutathione can virtually halt the progress of cataract development. I recommend 50 milligrams of glutathione a day.

Alpha lipoic acid

The reason that alpha lipoic acid works so well in concert with glutathione is that it helps to replace that antioxidant in the lens of the eye. Alpha lipoic acid is known as the universal antioxidant because it is both fat and water soluble. It can be absorbed by the fatty areas surrounding the optic nerve endings, and it can penetrate the water-soluble areas such as the eye lens. Therefore, it is a very important supplement for the protection of good vision. One hundred milligrams should be taken daily.

Quercetin

Quercetin is found in such foods as onions and apples and in some tea products. Its usefulness has been proven in decreasing cataracts, retinopathy and inflammation in the eye. It also counters mucus production, so it is helpful in the treatment of allergies, which often cause watery eyes. A dosage of 50 milligrams daily is sufficient.

Taurine

This amino acid is usually present in very high levels in the retina. It serves as a shield to the small nerve endings present in the macula that transmit the images from the eye to the brain, allowing us to see. If taurine is somehow depleted for whatever reason—genetics, poor diet or otherwise—the nerves are not properly shielded, and vision problems develop.

Interestingly, newborn babies do not have the ability to produce taurine right away, but they receive their supply from their mother's breast milk. If the mother decides to feed her infant with a prepared formula, it must contain taurine, or the baby will develop eye problems. Adults can supplement the taurine in their eyes by eating fish or other meat products, or by taking 100 milligrams per day in capsule form.

Vitamin C

For the treatment of glaucoma, 2 to 5 grams of vitamin C a day will significantly decrease the ocular pressure in the eye, reversing the progression of the disease and perhaps even preventing blindness.

Vitamin C protects so many parts of the body, but because it is water soluble, it is especially important to the health of the eye lens. Because the lens is not supplied by any blood vessels, any nutrients it gets must be able to disseminate through the liquid portion of the lens. Vitamin C is able to do so, and thus it is very important to the health of the eye. A dose of 300 to 500 milligrams is necessary for the prevention of cataracts. Long-term usage provides the best protection, so start now to reap the benefits of good vision later in life.

ASK DR. CHERRY

QUESTION: **Should I still wear sunglasses if I am taking these supplements to protect my vision?**

ANSWER: Absolutely! Any protection that can be given to the macula, the small area in the retina that is the sharpest focus of our vision, is welcome! Sunglasses that block 99 percent of the UVA and UVB rays are ideal. Natural supplements should not take the place of the first line of defense—the sunglasses. But neither should the sunglasses take the place of the supplements. Let the two work together to promote the health of your precious eyesight.

QUESTION: **What are antioxidants, and how can they protect my eyes?**

ANSWER: Antioxidants are a group of compounds that play a very protective role in your body. Their main purpose is to locate and neutralize a dangerous class of molecules known as free radicals. Free radicals are reactive substances that can do a great amount of damage to vital structures in your body, like cell membranes and DNA. Researchers now think that many of our most troubling modern diseases are either caused or worsened by free-radical damage.

Some free radicals are produced within your body as by-products of energy metabolism. If antioxidant levels in your body are adequate, you can usually handle this free-radical load. Unfortunately, today, most of us are exposed to higher than normal levels of free radicals in the forms of pollution, radiation and toxic chemicals in our air, food and water. At the same time, we're eating less fresh fruits and vegetables—the main sources of dietary antioxidants. This combination is a recipe for poor health and disease.

The eyes are particularly vulnerable to free-radical damage. Many serious eye diseases—like cataracts and macular degeneration—are thought to be associated with the effects of free radicals. For that reason, antioxidants such as lutein and zeaxanthin are important to the preservation of your vision and the protection of the delicate structure of your eyes.

ESSENTIAL NUTRIENTS TO PROTECT YOUR EYESIGHT

NUTRIENT	EFFECT	DAILY DOSAGE
Alpha lipoic acid	Antioxidant that regenerates vitamin C, vitamin E and glutathione—three powerful antioxidants that help defend the lens, macula and other eye tissues from free radicals	100 mg
Bilberry fruit powder	A natural source of anthocyanidins and flavonoids, both of which are powerful antioxidants that help reduce oxidative stress on the eyes	40 mg
Eyebright	Herb used to promote proper eye function and to ease over-sensitivity to light	10 mg
L-glutathione	Antioxidant that helps defend the lens, macula and other eye tissues from free radicals	50 mg
Lutein/zeaxanthin	The most biologically active carotenoids, especially important for promoting macular health	6 mg
Quercetin	Natural antioxidant flavonoid that helps protect the eyes from sun damage	50 mg
Taurine	Amino acid that has been shown to reduce oxidative damage to your eyes caused by sunlight, while stimulating your body's ability to remove waste by-products that accumulate in the retina	100 mg
Vitamin C	Essential vitamin and antioxidant that neutralizes free radicals in the lens, macula and other eye tissues	300–500 mg

CHAPTER 19

PROSTATE DISEASE

As the sun went down that evening, all the villagers who had any sick people in their homes, no matter what their diseases were, brought them to Jesus; and the touch of his hands healed every one!
—LUKE 4:40, TLB

M OST MEN SUFFER THE *PLAGUE* OF PROSTATE ENLARGEMENT AS THEY GROW OLDER. I call it a plague because the symptoms it causes bring such aggravation and misery, and the treatments offered by traditional medicine are just as unpleasant—at best. While it is a "natural" phenomenon for the prostate to enlarge with age, because the urethra runs directly through the middle of the prostate, any enlargement causes problems with urination—therein lies the misery. Doctors call this simple enlargement *benign prostatic hyperplasia,* or BPH, which indicates that the cells within the prostate have swollen. Four primary symptoms begin to occur in men who are developing an enlarged prostate gland—all of them unwelcome! Unfortunately, enlargement of the prostate is extremely common in men. Six out of ten men over the age of sixty develop prostate problems. By age seventy, 80 percent of men are displaying symptoms.[1]

Symptoms of Prostate Enlargement

The first thing that a man might notice is that it begins to take him longer to empty his bladder; his urination is slowing down. This indicates that the swelling prostate is pressing against the urethra and impeding the flow of urine. Second, it becomes harder to cut off the urinary stream, and this causes a dribbling problem that many men start to notice. Third, it becomes harder to start urinating in the first place, and finally, a man finds himself getting up in the night more and more frequently to use the bathroom. I have had patients who literally get up every thirty to forty-five minutes all through the night, every night, to go to the bathroom.

These symptoms can be very frustrating! Not only is it an embarrassing situation for a man, but add to that the fact that he begins to lose sleep, and you have a cause for other health problems due to the stress and sleep deprivation he experiences regularly.

Traditional Treatments Aren't Fun!

Generally, a man has to reach the point of absolute desperation before he agrees to some of the traditional treatments that are available for prostate enlargement. Many doctors will either freeze or burn out the prostate gland, neither of which is comfortable or pleasant for the patient. One newer, experimental treatment is to concentrate high frequency waves onto the prostate, in essence, to microwave it to try to shrink the tissue and alleviate the symptoms!

The most commonly used medical treatment for prostate enlargement is called the TURP. A man gets "turped" when he receives a *transurethral resection of the prostate,* a surgical procedure that slices into the prostate to reverse the inflammation. Most men don't want to submit themselves to the most unpleasant procedure of being "turped." But when symptoms worsen so that it is difficult to empty their bladder when they'd like, when they are getting up in the night every thirty or forty-five minutes or when they begin to suffer incontinence during the day, they are likely to submit to freezing, microwaving or being turped, just to get some relief!

Natural Treatments for
Prostate Enlargement

Fortunately, God has once again provided for the needs of His children.

Within the plant kingdom He has placed natural substances that have proven effective in relieving the symptoms of prostate enlargement, without having to undergo any of the treatments we've just discussed. Interestingly, the plants that produce these healing substances exist in many different parts of the world. For each culture, God has created "locally," unique compounds that provide relief for this very common and miserable condition.

These healing substances, when combined together, wield a potent punch against the symptoms of prostate enlargement. Let me caution you concerning your personal regimen for taking these natural substances. It is common for many people to practically overdose on a certain nutrient when they read that it might be helpful for their condition. The best thing to do, rather than taking just one substance and going overboard with it, is to properly combine them.

Think about how God set up His plant kingdom. He designed the chemicals within foods, but He never intended for us to just eat one food all of the time. We shouldn't eat just broccoli morning, noon and night, should we? God planned for us to have a balanced diet, and He spread out the nutrients through different foods for us to enjoy. As you learn to combine these natural remedies, you can watch the symptoms of prostate enlargement begin to disappear!

Saw palmetto

One of the most familiar treatments for the prostate gland is saw palmetto, which works in the body the same way as Proscar, an expensive medication sometimes prescribed to decrease inflammation in the prostate. Saw palmetto naturally inhibits the enzyme 5 alpha reductase, which causes some of the swelling that causes the symptoms. By reducing this inflammation, the prostate gland shrinks and the symptoms are reduced.

Men between the ages forty and fifty should take 320 milligrams per day, while men over the age of fifty should take 640 milligrams.

Pygeum

Numerous studies have been conducted that show the effectiveness of pygeum, when combined with saw palmetto, in reducing the symptoms of prostate disease.[2] Pygeum actually comes from a plum tree in Africa. A dose of 50 to 100 milligrams of pygeum extract per day is very helpful for men under the age of fifty. Men over fifty should take 200 milligrams a day.

Beta sitosterol

The sterols are a type of chemical compound that decreases inflammation. Beta sitosterol is especially effective in decreasing the swelling that occurs in the prostate; therefore, it is particularly good at increasing the urinary flow. Patients who begin taking beta sitosterol start getting up less and less frequently in the night to urinate. Getting a good night's sleep can make a huge difference in both a man's health and his mood.

Men between the ages of forty and fifty should take 12.5 milligrams per day, while men over the age of fifty should double the dosage to 25 milligrams per day.

Nettle root powder

While it may not sound like a smart idea to put something called *nettle root powder* into your body, nettle root powder has actually been used in many different countries as another potent anti-inflammatory. It not only contains the beta sitosterol we just discussed, but it also contains several other equally powerful sterols, which shrink the prostate and cause a decrease in the symptoms that men suffer.

Men between the ages of forty and fifty should take 150 milligrams per day, but men over the age of fifty should take 300 milligrams daily.

Rye pollen extract

Rye pollen extract has been used extensively in Europe for several decades. It works in two primary ways. Much like the other treatments we have discussed, it shrinks the prostate gland, bringing symptom relief, but additionally, it increases the force of bladder contractions. This helps a man begin to urinate when he needs to, and it prevents many of the dribbling problems that are such an annoyance.

Men between the ages of forty and fifty should take 189 milligrams per day, but men over the age of fifty should take the recommended dose of 378 milligrams daily.

Red clover and soy

Red clover and soy share similar properties due to a common compound they share, known as an *isoflavin*. In countries such as China where diets include a lot of soy, both prostate enlargement and prostate cancer are almost unheard of. Red clover actually has four different isoflavones, and soy has two, including the most common, *genistein*. But when red clover and soy are taken together, the combination of these isoflavins seems to provide protection from inflammation or other problems in the prostate.

Men between the ages of forty and fifty should take 80 milligrams of red clover blossom extract and 12.5 milligrams of soy isoflavones. Men over the age of fifty should double these dosages to 160 milligrams per day of red clover blossom extract and 25 milligrams of soy isoflavones.

Pumpkinseed extract

When men who consumed large amounts of pumpkinseeds began to notice an increase in their urinary flow, it was discovered that the sterol compounds within these seeds had an anti-inflammatory effect on the prostate gland. Now, fortunately, the benefits of the pumpkinseed can be achieved without actually having to eat a pumpkin full of seeds! The extract form is available and is just as effective in treating prostate problems. Men between the ages of forty and fifty should take 10 milligrams of pumpkinseed powder; men over the age of fifty should take 20 milligrams per day.

Seek Early Treatment!

So many men put off treating prostate enlargement because of fear or shame until they can hardly empty their bladders! When the condition reaches that point, they could easily end up needing to get "turped." But if the problem can be identified in its early stages, these natural treatments can eliminate the symptoms and the need for unnecessary and unpleasant medical intervention. Women, if your husbands have a prostate problem they are trying to ignore, encourage them to seek help early rather than late. Then begin taking these natural supplements right away!

God's natural provision is available, but it's up to us to begin to walk in the pathway to healing that He has for us. Pray about the problem, ask God what He would have you do, and then obey His instruction. There is no reason to continue suffering in misery. Begin today to find your pathway to healing of prostate problems.

🍒 ASK DR. CHERRY

QUESTION: **What is a PSA level, and what does it indicate?**

ANSWER: A PSA level indicates the level of inflammation that is occurring within the prostate gland and can be an indicator of prostate cancer. PSA actually stands for "prostate specific antigen." The levels of this antigen increase as the prostate enlarges, when prostate infection occurs or with prostate cancer. A reading over 4 means that the prostate is enlarged and medical intervention of some kind should take place before further problems occur.

QUESTION: **Is there a certain form of saw palmetto extract that I should take in order to prevent prostate enlargement?**

ANSWER: In the world of nutritional supplements, not all herbs are created equal. In its natural state, saw palmetto contains about 1.5 percent of an oily substance believed to be the active component that helps support healthy prostate function. This is a very low concentration that would require taking enormous quantities to get the beneficial effects.

Fortunately, special methods can be used to create a concentrated extract of saw palmetto with a much higher percentage of the active component. With this high concentration, much less needs to be taken. In fact, clinical studies that have proven the benefits of saw palmetto for the prostate have all used concentrated extracts of the herb.[3] Therefore, products that provide saw palmetto in its low-potency state cannot give you the same benefits that are seen in the scientific studies.

ESSENTIAL NUTRIENTS TO AVOID PROSTATE PROBLEMS

NATURAL SUBSTANCE	EFFECT	DOSAGE FOR AGE 40–50	DOSAGE FOR AGE 50+
Saw palmetto berry extract	Herb rich in lipids and phytosterols that promote healthy dihydrotestosterone (DHT) levels in the prostate	320 mg	640 mg
Pygeum bark extract	Herb that supports normal hormone levels in the prostate	100 mg	200 mg
Beta sitosterol	Natural plant sterol that promotes healthy DHT levels in the prostate	12.5 mg	25 mg
Soy isoflavones	Source of two key isoflavones—genistein and diadzein—that promote healthy DHT levels in the prostate	12.5 mg	25 mg
Rye pollen extract	Herbal extract containing compounds that promote healthy DHT levels in the prostate	189 mg	378 mg
Nettle root powder	Herb that is a rich source of many phytonutrients—like sterols and lignans—that support healthy prostate function	150 mg	300 mg
Red clover blossom extract	Herb rich in isoflavones that promote healthy hormone levels in the prostate	80 mg	160 mg
Pumpkinseed powder	Natural source of zinc and other nutrients known to be beneficial for healthy prostate tissue	10 mg	20 mg

CHAPTER 20

SYMPTOMS OF MENOPAUSE

*Now a woman, having a flow of blood for twelve
years, who had spent all of her livelihood on
physicians and could not be healed by any, came
from behind and touched the border of His garment.
And immediately her flow of blood stopped.*

—LUKE 8:43–44, NKJV

JESUS LOVED WOMEN. When our Lord walked on the earth, He elevated the status of women, spending quality time with them, ministering to them and eventually giving them responsibilities and an important position in His church.

Jesus was concerned about the problems that women face. A very touching incident is described in the eighth chapter of Luke. One day a woman with an issue of blood approached Him for healing. Most likely, her medical problem was a female one, and the Bible tells us that she had "suffered many things of many physicians" (Mark 5:26). But when she touched Jesus, power flowed from His body into hers, and she was healed.

How important it is for us to turn to Jesus and find the healing pathway that He has planned for us! This woman had suffered under medical treatments that did not cure her, but when she turned to Jesus in her desperation, she received the healing she so desperately needed. And when Jesus realized who it was who touched Him for healing, He commended her faith (Mark 5:34).

God is still concerned about the needs of women today. All women who experience the length of life that God has promised them will pass through the phase of *menopause,* which signals a drop in estrogen levels and cessation of fertility. In my clinical research, I find that nearly forty-nine hundred women a day enter menopause in this country alone. Menopause is a natural process, but especially in the United States, it has become fraught with aggravating symptoms that are difficult to deal with, not to mention the increased possibility of contracting several devastating diseases.

Suffering at the Hands of Doctors

In the early 1900s most women would only live to the age of forty-seven or forty-eight, and so menopause was a very rare occurrence. Women simply didn't live long enough to go through it! But as the life span of women began to increase, doctors began seeing certain symptoms appearing in aging women: hot flashes, mood swings, depression, anxiety and sleeplessness. Unfortunately, these symptoms were grossly misunderstood by the medical community.

When a woman who was sitting in a perfectly cool room suddenly broke out into a sweat, or when she sobbed uncontrollably for days at a time, doctors diagnosed it as the only thing they understood it to be: insanity. Many menopausal women were hospitalized in psychiatric units simply for displaying what we consider "normal" symptoms that greet women as they grow older.

Fortunately, in the early 1960s, doctors began to understand that menopausal symptoms were caused by the body's ceasing to produce the hormone estrogen. Synthetic, artificial estrogen was then offered to women to alleviate the menopausal symptoms, and amazingly, the hot flashes, the night sweats and the mood swings all disappeared. But then a startling problem began to take place: Uterine cancer rates began to skyrocket. Some statistics even show a leap of 13 to 15 percent in women who took prescription estrogen! Eventually, doctors discovered that adding progestin to the estrogen that women were taking helped protect the uterine lining and decrease the risk of uterine cancer. But then the risk of breast cancer seemed to leap sky high.

Now it is important to stress that most doctors are motivated by the desire to help people, but without God's help, they are limited in what they understand and in their ability to help. So it is true that many women have suffered at their hands. When we begin to understand that medical treatments cure hot flashes but cause cancer, it is time to seek God for a better way.

Symptoms of Menopause

The most obvious problems that women encounter when they reach a certain age actually begin before menopause, involving the cessation of the menstrual cycle, takes place. The phase in which symptoms occur before menopause is called the *perimenopausal* period. These symptoms can be quite aggravating!

One of the first symptoms will be irregular periods. A woman may have two or three normal periods, and then skip one or two, or a period may come at an unexpected time. Then she may notice stranger symptoms: Hot flashes and night sweats are among the most common. She may not be aware of more subtle changes that are taking place: Vascular changes in the eye begin to cause a fuzziness in the vision. Forgetfulness, mood swings, anxiety and difficulty concentrating signal that hormonal changes are happening. Many women experience a crawling sensation on their skin, like an insect is crawling on their arm, but when they look, there is nothing there. Urinary tract infections increase as vaginal dryness increases. And one especially troubling symptom that is caused by a decrease in the female hormones is an increasing loss of scalp hair, along with the development of hair in other parts of their body.

Diseases Associated With Menopause

While these symptoms are very annoying to women, they aren't particularly life threatening. However, there are several diseases that often accompany menopause, which are far more serious.

Osteoporosis

Osteoporosis, in which a woman's bones become porous-like and brittle, is perhaps the most well-known disease associated with menopause. Statistics concerning osteoporosis are alarming. By the time half of all women reach the age of sixty, osteoporosis becomes evident on their x-rays. By the time a woman reaches eighty years of age, she could easily have lost almost half of her bone mass *and not even be aware of it!* The most frequent clue that alerts a woman to the fact that she has osteoporosis is a fracture of some sort, perhaps a broken hip or a broken leg.

Many times, a woman may think she was injured as the result of a fall, but what happens in many cases is that the fall is actually the result of the injury. A woman may be walking along, and because her bones have become so ravaged by the disease, her hipbone will break, or the bones in her leg will snap, and that is what actually causes her fall. You can imagine how easily it would be for this to take place if a woman has lost almost half of her bone mass!

Estrogen has been proven to halt the progression of osteoporosis and even reverse the disease, especially when it is combined with calcium and vitamin D. But as I have already mentioned, with prescription estrogen, the incidences of breast cancer skyrocket. However, in Asia, both osteoporosis and breast cancer are virtually unheard of, and the differences in their diet, as we will discuss, hold the key for our own health in this area.

Heart disease

Among women between the ages of forty-five and sixty-four, one woman in nine will develop heart disease, but over the age of sixty-five, that number triples to one in three! It seems that women are protected from heart disease in their younger years, but by the time they reach their sixties, they have caught up with men in the risk of developing heart problems. Heart disease is actually the number one killer of women.

Breast cancer

Breast cancer is becoming a concern for more and more women, especially as the number of diagnosed cases has increased dramatically. Prescription-dispensed estrogen and progestin, while providing relief from most of the other symptoms of menopause, have caused skyrocketing rates of breast cancer, as we mentioned.

What are women to do? Modern medicine seems to be offering only two choices: Either suffer through the often miserable symptoms that menopause brings, or put yourself at a much greater risk of developing a deadly disease such as uterine or breast cancer. Fortunately, God's health plan offers a better option!

Natural Substances Every
Woman Should Take

Man cannot duplicate the benefits of God's creation. There are basic substances found in nature that have been proven to provide relief for women who are experiencing hormonal changes in their bodies. They also serve to protect women from developing the deadly diseases we discussed as they grow older. Symptom relief and protection from disease—all in one package, without any known side effects! That is God's pathway for a long and satisfying life for women.

Soy and red clover

The isoflavones present in soy and red clover, shown to be beneficial for prostate enlargement in men, have amazing properties for women as well. Soy, especially as an ingredient in tofu and miso, is an important part of Asian women's regular diet. This is a primary reason why so many Asian women do not experience the terrible symptoms of menopause that most American women do. Soy has two primary isoflavins, genistein being the most prominent, and red clover has four, so when these two are taken in combination with each other, the results are powerful.

While soy mimics the diet of most Asian cultures, red clover contains many of the properties of the legumes found in Mediterranean countries, such as beans and chickpeas. In both of these cultures, menopausal symptoms, osteoporosis and breast cancer are virtually unheard of.

In addition, soy is what is called a "selective estrogen receptor modulator," which simply means that it blocks the receptor sites that would generally bind with the prescription estrogen and cause either breast or uterine cancer. Studies show that women who are taking higher doses of soy isoflavones demonstrate a 54 percent decrease in uterine cancer.[1] The same is true of heart disease.[2]

The FDA has begun to allow soy to make a "heart protective claim," based on the many studies that show its role in decreasing the LDL (bad) cholesterol and increasing the HDL (good) cholesterol levels. Also, the genistein present in both soy and red clover inhibits the breakdown of bone in the body and stimulates the formation of new bone. Amazingly, soy and red clover provide powerful symptom relief from menopause and, unlike traditional medical treatments, do not cause breast or uterine cancer or heart problems. In fact, they actually *protect* women from these diseases!

Fifty milligrams daily of the soy isoflavones and 500 milligrams daily of red clover leaf extract will bring the greatest benefit.

Black cohosh

When a woman needs symptom relief, she generally needs it *now,* if not *yesterday!* Black cohosh, a phytoestrogen (estrogen derived from a plant), begins to show results within *two weeks time!* This herb comes from a buttercup plant that was used for centuries by the American Indians to relieve menopausal symptoms. The chemicals within the black cohosh also, like the soy and red clover, bind to the receptor sites and help to prevent uterine or breast cancer.

There are no known side effects whatsoever for those who take black cohosh as a supplement; it is one of the safest but most potent herbs available. I have found a significant improvement in symptoms in nearly 100 percent of the women who took it. Black cohosh seems to alleviate headaches, heart palpitations, depression and anxiety, and vaginal dryness, thus preventing urinary tract infections. It also alleviates dizziness, high blood pressure and blood sugar.

A dose of 80 milligrams per day is recommended.

Dong quai (angelica)

Dong quai is an Asian herb that is most helpful when combined with the other treatments we are discussing. Its primary benefits are associated with stopping the hot flashes and vaginal dryness. A dose of 300 milligrams per day is best.

Ginseng

Having been used for centuries all over the world, ginseng is used primarily as a treatment for stress. Siberian ginseng will improve the mood and stress relief of a woman, especially when her hormone levels begin to drop off as she grows older. The recommended dose is 200 milligrams a day.

Boron

Boron is a mineral that helps the body absorb calcium and therefore proves helpful in strengthening bone structure and protecting women from osteoporosis. Boron should be taken at a dose of 3 milligrams per day.

Bromelain

Bromelain is helpful to the body for a number of reasons. It is primarily an anti-inflammatory, so therefore it helps to prevent blood clots from forming, as well as providing relief from arthritis and other joint problems. In women facing menopause, it is especially helpful in curbing the edema, or swelling, caused by fluid retention. The recommended dose is 45 milligrams per day.

These substances are, I believe, just the beginning of our discovery of the relief God has already provided to women suffering from the terrible symptoms of menopause. In America, it is estimated that 55 to 60 percent of all women will have significant problems in this area as they age, but amazingly, as of this writing, over four hundred estrogen compounds have been discovered in nature. God's way is to provide relief from the symptoms and, at the same time, provide protection from diseases such as osteoporosis and heart disease. What a healing God we serve! You don't have to suffer through menopause anymore! Begin to trust Him today to reveal the pathway to healing He has just for you.

ASK DR. CHERRY

QUESTION: **Do the natural substances you have listed as beneficial for menopausal women have any benefit at all for men?**

ANSWER: It is interesting to consider that all men are, in fact, part women, and all women are part men. Both men and women produce the hormones estrogen and testosterone, but what makes the difference is the prominence of one or the other in a person. In women, estrogen is prominent, and this causes the body changes that make a woman "female." Testosterone is what makes a man "male."

A new treatment that is being developed for prostate cancer in men is to give them a dose of artificial estrogen to offset the testosterone in their bodies. It is interesting to consider that God provides protection for both men and women from two of their biggest killers—prostate cancer and breast cancer—through the same means: the four hundred estrogen compounds that have been placed in nature.

QUESTION: **Do I need to take the nutrients you have suggested if I am already undergoing hormone replacement therapy?**

ANSWER: Many women find that taking the nutritional supplements recommended in this chapter, along with eating a good diet and getting daily exercise, is all they need to help them through this life transition.

Other women may be taking hormone replacement therapy (HRT) on the advice of their doctor. HRT usually consists of a combination of synthetic estrogen (Premarin) and progesterone (Provera). While these drugs can be helpful in reducing menopausal symptoms and in warding off osteoporosis (brittle bones), they also have potential side effects, such as bloating, irritability and headaches. Also, HRT may increase your risk for breast cancer and blood clots. Because of these risks, the pros and cons of HRT should be discussed carefully with your doctor.

The question of whether or not to combine a nutritional supplement program with HRT is also a question for your doctor.

QUESTION: **How can I deal with the hot flashes I am experiencing during menopause?**

ANSWER: If you are having hot flashes associated with menopause, the following tips may bring you some relief:

- When a hot flash starts, go somewhere that is cool.
- Sleeping in a cooler room may keep hot flashes from waking you up during the night.
- Dress in layers that you can take off if you get warm.
- Use sheets and clothing that let your skin "breathe."
- Try having a cold drink (water or juice) at the beginning of a hot flash.

ESSENTIAL NUTRIENTS TO EASE THE DISCOMFORTS OF MENOPAUSE

NATURAL SUBSTANCE	EFFECT	DAILY DOSAGE
Red clover leaf extract	Herb rich in isoflavones that helps balance hormones, promote healthy bones and support cardiovascular function	500 mg
Dong quai root extract	Herb traditionally used to support hormonal balance in women	300 mg
Siberian ginseng root extract	Member of the ginseng family traditionally used in both China and Russia to help increase resistance to stress, fatigue and illness	200 mg
Black cohosh root extract	Herb rich in phytosterols that has been used traditionally to help support hormonal balance in women	80 mg

NATURAL SUBSTANCE	EFFECT	DAILY DOSAGE
Soy isoflavones	Natural compounds from soy that help regulate hormone balance and support skeletal and cardiovascular health	50 mg
Bromelain	Enzyme derived from pineapple that helps with the digestion and absorption of nutrients	45 mg
Boron	Mineral that helps strengthen bones and cartilage	3 mg

CHAPTER 21

PMS: Stopping the Monthly Plague

*He personally carried away our sins in his own body
on the cross so we can be dead to sin and live for
what is right. You have been healed by his wounds!*
—1 PETER 2:24, NLT

WOMEN DO NOT HAVE TO SUFFER FROM PMS SYMPTOMS. As many as 85 percent of women suffer from one or more symptoms of premenstrual syndrome (PMS), according to the most recent set of guidelines released by the American College of Obstetricians and Gynecologists.[1] The most common complaints seem to center around mood symptoms such as irritability, anxiety or depression that occur in the week or two before menstruation.

Many women suddenly find themselves weeping, screaming with anger and frustration or feeling unusually tense with no real external cause. Although the exact causes for premenstrual syndrome are not fully understood, researchers suspect that they are the result of a hormonal imbalance and an increased sensitivity to those unbalanced hormones.

The end result of the hormone imbalance is a lowered level of the brain chemical neurotransmitter *serotonin*. Some studies indicate that in women who suffer PMS, the ratio of estrogen to progesterone tends to be higher than in women who are free of PMS symptoms. Certain lifestyle changes are recommended to all women who suffer from PMS, such as decreasing caffeine intake and increasing exercise levels.

Natural Supplements Can Help

Data are beginning to accumulate on the value of certain supplements as effective treatments for PMS.

Calcium

For years, doctors have observed one interesting association that has not been understood. Women who suffered from PMS when they were younger had a much higher risk of developing osteoporosis as they grew older. As it turns out, calcium is probably the common deficiency in both premenstrual syndrome and osteoporosis. Not surprisingly, then, calcium supplements are an effective treatment for the troubling symptoms of PMS.

The most convincing data on the benefits of supplements for PMS consistently point to calcium supplementation. Women who take 1,000 to 1,200 milligrams of calcium daily have a significant reduction in premenstrual symptoms. We currently recommend that women (and men as well) supplement their diets with a total of 1,000 milligrams of calcium in four different forms—the citrate, carbonate, ascorbate and gluconate forms. All of these can be combined and taken in a basic nutrient supplement. Remember, however, it is the citrate form that is the most easily absorbed of all the calcium supplements.

Vitamins and minerals

Some studies have also suggested benefits in taking supplements of magnesium at a dose of 400 milligrams daily and vitamin E at a dose of 800 international units (in its natural form) daily. Vitamin B_6 has also been widely used for PMS; especially due to its preventive benefits against stroke and heart disease, I recommend taking it at a dose of 75 milligrams a day.

Chasteberry

One herbal supplement that can be very useful in alleviating symptoms of premenstrual syndrome is the herb *vitex,* also known as *chasteberry.* Decreased PMS symptoms were noted in 70 to 80 percent of the women who used this herbal supplement, which tends to increase the levels of progesterone in the body in a natural way.[2] Simply follow the directions on the bottle if you sense that God is leading you to try chasteberry.

God created the female body, and He knows exactly how it functions in all its intricacy. If you are suffering the terrible symptoms of PMS, if it is making you miserable—along with everyone around you—begin to pray and seek God's wisdom as to what path He would have you take to find relief. You don't have to waste one single day to cramps, irritable moods or discomfort! Begin to pray specifically for the serotonin levels within your brain, that they would come into balance, along with the levels of estrogen and progesterone in your body. Pray for the successful absorption of the necessary vitamins and minerals to help ease your symptoms.

Don't stop at just bringing the problem before the Father in prayer. Do what things you can do naturally to take care of the situation. I recommend that you try the following:

- Get enough rest.

- Try to reduce your stress levels, especially when you sense the onset of symptoms.

- Take a hot bath to ease the cramps.

- Exercise consistently.

- Cut back on the caffeine.

- Begin taking supplements of the vitamins and nutrients I have outlined in this chapter.

Once you have done all that you know to do in following your pathway to healing, stand in faith for it, and expect God to keep His promise.

ASK DR. CHERRY

QUESTION: **What effect does calcium have on PMS symptoms?**

ANSWER: Calcium helps to alleviate symptoms of premenstrual syndrome by aiding the body in balancing proper hormone levels.

QUESTION: **I have heard about the condition called pre-menstrual dysphoria disorder. Can you explain what it is?**

ANSWER: When PMS presents with certain specific depressive symptoms, psychiatrists sometimes classify it as premenstrual dysphoria disorder.

CHAPTER 22

REVERSING THE
EFFECTS OF
VARICOSE VEINS

For the life of the flesh is in the blood.
—LEVITICUS 17:11

GOD DEVISED A UNIQUE AND INCREDIBLE SYSTEM, DEFYING GRAVITY, TO RETURN BLOOD FROM OUR LOWER EXTREMITIES TO THE HEART. Our physical movement (walking, running, climbing and so forth) in this physical world is dependent on proper blood flow. The heart pumps the blood through the arteries into the lower extremities—supplying nutrients along the way—and then returns the venous blood up the leg and back to the heart, literally defying the laws of gravity.

God's marvelous design can be seen in a series of one-way valves in the veins that allow blood to flow in only one direction—upward toward the heart instead of downward toward the ground. Blood is literally squeezed up the veins of the lower extremities by the contraction of muscles in the leg.

Many people notice swelling in their lower extremities after they have been sitting for long periods of time, such as at a desk or when traveling by car or airplane. They have not contracted these muscles in order to help circulation. Even minor contractions of the calf muscles while sitting—raising the foot and rotating the ball of the foot, for example—is sufficient to return blood back up the leg to the heart. However, if blood is allowed to accumulate in the lower extremities (a condition known as *venous stasis*), the risk of blood pooling and, potentially, blood clotting is greatly increased. This can become a serious problem, particularly if it involves the deep veins of the leg.

One of the problems of our modern culture is decreased physical activity and a sedentary lifestyle, which puts us more at risk for blood pooling. Even though this condition does not usually lead to the formation of blood clots, it does increase the pressure in the veins. This increased pressure can break down the one-way valves designed to carry blood back to the heart. When this happens, the vessels below the valves swell, causing what we know as *varicose veins*.

Varicose veins cause fluid to accumulate in the lower extremities (edema), change the skin color and, in severe cases, cause ulceration. Leg pain, tiredness in the lower extremities and itching can follow. Doctors refer to this problem as *chronic venous insufficiency* (CVI). It occurs in 10 to 15 percent of males and 20 to 25 percent of females.

The conventional treatment for this condition has been the use of support stockings (which provide compression), accompanied by periodic elevation of the legs to relieve pressure in the veins. Occasionally, doctors will recommend vascular surgery, such as vein stripping or sclerotherapy.

Natural Therapy God's Way

In His infinite wisdom, God has provided an herbal product for us through the plant kingdom that has shown great promise in treating this annoying and potentially serious problem of varicose veins. The extract is from horse chestnut seed (*aesculus hippocastanum*). The common name of "horse chestnut seed" was given because the seeds resemble a horse's eyes.

Reports date back into the 1800s of the use of horse chestnut seed extract for the treatment of venous disease and varicose veins. Scientists are just now beginning to study this herbal treatment and its effect on varicose veins. They have now identified many of the active beneficial chemicals that God placed within this plant. The primary function of the chemicals in horse chestnut extract is to reduce fluid loss from capillaries, which results from increased pressure in the veins. Research shows that the extract can help stop enzymes that weaken the walls of capillaries and improve circulation by increasing the flexibility of the blood vessels, which in turn improves blood flow.[1]

These chemicals prevent edema and swelling. Studies have shown that they can increase the tone of the veins and help prevent leakage from the capillaries. Study results show a reduction in the swelling in the legs and significant improvements in such problems as itching, pain and the feeling of fullness in the lower extremities. The horse chestnut extract is safe and well tolerated, as demonstrated by the results of numerous studies, some of which involved over five thousand patients.[2]

The extract is available in tablet or capsule form. In fact, a major pharmaceutical company in the United States has introduced a product known as Venastat, made from horse chestnut extract, to promote leg vein health. This is commercially available and is taken in a dosage of 48 milligrams twice daily.

If you suffer from varicose veins, it is often helpful to raise your feet at or above the level of your heart for at least forty-five minutes at the end of each day to take pressure off of the veins.

AUTHOR'S NOTE: If you have renal or kidney problems, you should use caution in taking any kind of herbal medicines since all orally ingested chemicals go through the liver and are filtered by the kidneys. In the case of varicose veins, I would urge you, as always, to consult with a physician who is familiar with both natural as well as conventional treatments.

ASK DR. CHERRY

QUESTION: **I've heard that people with varicose veins should wear support hose. Is that true?**

ANSWER: I usually recommend that patients with varicose veins use support hosiery during their waking hours as well as taking the horse chestnut extract. The correct support hose are knee-high compressive or elastic stockings that squeeze the blood up through the veins with each small muscle contractions.

QUESTION: **Are varicose veins ever serious?**

ANSWER: Varicose veins themselves are not a serious condition, but they could be associated with a potentially life-threatening disease known as *acute thrombophlebitis.* Be sure to have a physician check for the presence of this disease if you are exhibiting symptoms of varicose veins. Acute thrombophlebitis needs prompt medical attention, which includes blood-thinning measures. It is imperative that it be treated carefully by a physician. The horse chestnut extract should only be used in situations of chronic venous insufficiency and valve breakdown.

CHAPTER 23

NEW HOPE FOR PREVENTING BREAST CANCER

For God has not given us a spirit of fear, but of
power and of love and of a sound mind.
—2 TIMOTHY 1:7, NKJV

THE WORDS *BREAST CANCER* STRIKE FEAR INTO NEARLY EVERY WOMAN WHO HEARS THEM. But, according to Scripture, God did not give us a spirit of fear. As believers, we do not have to live in dread of contracting a life-threatening disease. God promises us a spirit of power, of love and of a sound, or disciplined, mind. As we pursue His pathway of health and healing, we can be free from fear of disease.

Although over 180,000 new cases of breast cancer will be diagnosed this year, and one woman in eight will develop breast cancer over the course of a normal life span, it does not have to strike the child of God. We are not to be frightened or discouraged over these statistics; we have power against this disease through God's revelation knowledge. We not only have spiritual authority through Christ as believers, but we also have God's healing provision in the plant kingdom that will give us power over breast cancer.

Twelve Natural Preventive Measures

The National Cancer Institute has estimated that simply making changes in dietary intake might prevent 60 to 70 percent of breast cancer cases. What follows are the top twelve ways you can keep yourself from becoming a breast cancer statistic.

1. Eat that tofu!

The incidence of breast cancer in Asia, the Mediterranean countries and numerous other areas in the world are very low. Researchers believe the low rates of breast cancer are due, in large part, to the intake of soy products, as we have mentioned. More recently, as Asians began following a Western-type diet, their incidence of breast cancer rose steadily. The phytoestrogens, known as isoflavones, in soy are actually cancer preventives. These isoflavones bind to estrogen receptor sites and actually guard against the development of breast cancer.

Soy products contain other natural chemicals such as *protease inhibitors,* which prevent cancer-promoting genes from being activated, and *saponins,* which can keep cancer cells from multiplying.

Soy can be obtained as a soy-protein powder and used in drinks; soy flour is also available. Of course, the traditional soy dishes—such as tofu—are very healthful, although I have never been a big tofu fan. Soy products that are fortified with calcium can help prevent breast cancer cells from multiplying and dividing. You might consider trying soy milk on cereal.

2. Take red clover extract.

Perhaps an even better source of these beneficial isoflavones is an extract derived from red clover. Red clover contains four major isoflavones that, when taken daily, appear to be a promising and effective method for women to protect their bodies against the potential of breast cancer.

3. Eat lots of fish.

Study after study demonstrates that women who eat more fish have lower rates of breast cancer. Part of this protection comes from omega-3 fatty acids that are found in fish such as salmon, cod, mackerel, herring, sardines and trout. The omega-3 fatty acids are really oils that the human body can convert to a chemical known as *prostaglandins*. Certain types of protective prostaglandins keep breast cells from multiplying and dividing.

Patients with a strong family history of breast cancer or unusually thick breasts with increased amounts of fibrous tissue might want to consider taking omega-3 capsules daily. A study published in the *Journal of the*

National Cancer Institute found that taking fish oil capsules increased the concentration of omega-3 fatty acids (EPA and DHA) in breast tissue. Some natural sources are canola oil, walnuts and flaxseed.

4. Avoid cooking with corn oil.

Certain types of oils, such as saturated fats and other vegetable oils containing omega-6 fatty acids, may actually promote breast cancer. Polyunsaturated oils, like corn oil, may contribute to this also.

5. Add kiwi fruit to your diet.

The *Journal of the American College of Nutrition* ranked kiwi fruit as the most nutrient-dense of all fruits, providing vitamin E, magnesium and potassium and also proving to be a good source of dietary fiber. Kiwi provides twice as much vitamin C as an orange! Studies show that vitamin C can inhibit breast cell division, thus reducing the risk of breast cancer.

6. Eat ten almonds and five prunes a day.

For some time, we have recommended adding nuts to your daily dietary intake. Approximately ten salt-free almonds a day can offer numerous health benefits. Because they are a rich source of vitamin E, they also play an important role in preventing breast cancer.

Laboratory studies show that vitamin E decreases the incidence of mammary tumors that form after exposure to cancer-causing substances. It actually prevented the cancer cells from developing and provided a killing effect on the cells after they developed.

Personally, I like to combine the almonds I eat each day with five prunes. Prunes have turned out to be a medical "super fruit" in the fight against cancer. Because of the prune's remarkable ability to absorb oxygen-free radicals, they may also help retard the aging process in the body, especially in the brain.

7. Go orange.

There are some unique chemicals contained in citrus fruits, and especially in oranges, that fight breast cancer. *Hesperetin* and *naringenin* both prevent cancer cell division and also help neutralize cancer-causing chemicals in the body. Another chemical found in oranges, *limonene,* has potent cancer-fighting properties.

8. Take psyllium.

Add 1 tablespoon of psyllium to your diet daily, and you can further lower your risk of breast cancer. Women who eat more dietary fiber have a lower risk of breast cancer than those who eat a less amount of fiber. Consumption of psyllium and wheat bran results in a much lower rate of tumor development. You can buy psyllium husks or orange-flavored psyllium supplements (which I prefer) and use them daily in your diet.

9. Fiber, fiber, fiber

Fibers, such as wheat bran, tend to bind cancer-causing agents in the gastrointestinal tract and keep them from being absorbed. While psyllium is one good source of fiber, there are others. These sources of fiber include fruits and vegetables in general, and particularly in the skin or peels of fruits such as apples. Pinto beans are also a good fiber source, as are kidney beans. When shopping for flour or bread products, look for whole-wheat products.

10. Eat cabbage and broccoli.

God created a unique chemical compound, indole-3-carbinol, that reduces the body's production of certain types of estrogen leading to breast cancer. I found that these indoles also stop human breast cancer cells dead in their tracks. To reap the benefits of this protective substance, you should eat plenty of cabbage, broccoli and brussels sprouts.

11. Stock up on yogurt.

Yogurt contains high amounts of calcium, which can inhibit the division of breast cancer cells. Yogurt also stimulates gamma interferon, which helps fight cancer by enhancing the function of the immune system.

12. Take vitamin A.

Beta carotene is the best source of vitamin A. A dose of 15 milligrams daily as a supplement is recommended. Studies consistently show that populations that consume the most vitamin A have the lowest levels of breast cancer.

❥ ASK DR. CHERRY

Q UESTION: **I have heard that hormone replacement therapy can cause breast cancer. Is this true?**

A NSWER: When doctors began to treat menopausal women with prescription estrogen, the rates of uterine cancer rose alarmingly. Doctors eventually learned to counter that effect by combining prescription estrogen with progestin, but then the incidences of breast cancer rose sky high. Studies now show that prescription-dispensed estrogen and progestin, while providing relief from most of the other symptoms of menopause, put women at risk for breast cancer. Fortunately God has placed natural remedies within the plant kingdom that can help women through that transition phase of their lives without the residual risk of developing cancer.

Q UESTION: **If I should not use corn oil for cooking, is there an alternative that I should use?**

A NSWER: Yes, there is! Cook instead with olive oil. Olive oil contains monounsaturated fats, which have great heart benefits as well as cancer-preventive benefits. The oleic and steric acids in olive oil help reduce the risk of breast cancer. Olive oil can be used alone on salads or mixed with vinegar as a simple dressing.

CHAPTER 24

THE FALLACY OF FAD DIETS

*Bless the LORD, O my soul, and forget not all His
benefits…Who satisfies your mouth with good
things, so that your youth is renewed like the eagle's.*
—PSALM 103:2, 5, NKJV

IT'S NO SECRET THAT THE GENERAL AMERICAN PUBLIC IS INCREASINGLY
MORE OVERWEIGHT. In fact, there seems to be a direct correlation in the
last decade or so between the size of our cars (sport utility vehicles), the
size of our meals ("Could you super-size that?") and the size of our waist-
lines! In 1980, 46 percent of adults in the United States age twenty or
older were overweight or obese; by 1999, the number had increased to 60
percent.

We all know that it's not good to be overweight. But it's not just a matter
of how we look. Did you know that being just ten to twenty pounds overweight increases your risk of premature death? Those excess pounds
increase your risk of heart disease, diabetes, cancer, asthma and other illnesses. In fact, every two-pound increase in weight increases the risk of
arthritis by at least 9 percent, and a woman who gains more than twenty
pounds after age eighteen doubles her risk of postmenopausal breast
cancer. I have found a weight gain of *just eleven pounds* will *double* the risk
of acquiring type 2 diabetes!

Are You Overweight and at Risk for Disease?

A person's body mass index (BMI) and waist circumference are two useful indicators for determining whether you are at increased risk for health problems associated with being overweight or obese. Generally, the higher your BMI (your height to weight ratio) the higher your health risk, and the risk increases if your waist size is greater than thirty-five inches for women or forty inches for men.

Calculate your own risk

To find out if you are overweight and to determine your health risk, first find your BMI by using the following formula:

(Your weight [in pounds] x 704.5) divided by (your height [in inches] x your height [in inches])

For example, someone who is 5'6" (or 66 inches) and weighs 195 pounds would calculate their BMI as follows: BMI = (195 x 704.5) divided by (66 x 66) = 31.5

Use the final answer (that is, 31.5) to apply to the chart below to measure your health risk relative to normal weight:[1]

BMI		WAIST LESS THAN OR EQUAL TO 35" (WOMEN) OR 40" (MEN)	WAIST GREATER THAN 35" (WOMEN) OR 40" (MEN)
18.5 or less	Underweight	Low risk	Low risk
18.6–24.9	Normal	Low risk	Low risk
25.0–29.9	Overweight	Increased risk	High risk
30.0–34.9	Obese	High risk	Very high risk
35.0–39.9	Obese	Very high risk	Very high risk
40.0 or greater	Extremely obese	Extremely high risk	Extremely high risk

If you think you need to start dieting, you are not alone. The public's awareness of this widening problem (no pun intended!) has increased dramatically in the last several years, as evidenced by the number of fad diets being promoted almost every time you turn on the television set. People want to lose the weight! I estimate that at any given time 40 percent of women and 30 percent of men are on some sort of diet. But just who has the right plan? Is the new concept of "low-carb, high-fat" diets really a dream come true? Or is a low-fat diet the answer?

Finding the true solution that will work for you requires cutting through the confusion that is presently in the public forum on this issue and taking a look at the facts. Let's consider some of the most popular diets that are on the market today.

Popular "Fad" Diets

The age-old theme of "eat less and exercise more" hasn't been popular enough to launch any diet book onto the bestseller list. What does sell, however, is any book that promises some new "miracle" or "breakthrough" method for easy weight loss. While there may be one or two good points about each of the new, popular fad diets on the market today, by and large, they don't produce long-term results. They may even prove to be risky to your health rather than beneficial.

Most of these diets are based on the principle of monitoring two metabolic hormones, insulin and glucagon, and the regulation of glucose, the blood sugar that all carbohydrates will eventually become. Because the brain needs glucose to survive, there must be a certain amount of it present at all times. However, because high blood glucose levels (hyperglycemia) are damaging to the body, insulin, which decreases blood glucose, and glucagon, which increases it, regulate the levels.

After you eat a meal, glucose floods the bloodstream and the pancreas secretes insulin, which brings the blood glucose levels back down to normal. Glucagon has the opposite effect: If blood glucose levels get too low, it will signal the release of glucose from other storage sites (primarily the liver) to keep the brain in a full supply. This happens frequently at night when you are sleeping. Because you go for several hours without eating, the supply of glucose for the brain must come from somewhere within the body, which the glucagon works to supply.

Another concept important for understanding the major diet books is the glycemic index. This index measures how quickly certain foods (carbohydrates) are digested and become present in the bloodstream as glucose.

Foods such as white bread, pure sugar, pasta and potatoes are more quickly digested (higher glycemic index) than foods such as beans or wheat bread. The proposed problem with foods with a higher glycemic index is that they can cause a rapid rise in glucose and a greater insulin response in the body. However, the glycemic index only accounts for foods eaten isolated from each other, not those eaten together in a meal.

Armed with these facts, you will be able to understand the functioning principles of the following dietary regimens.

Dr. Atkins' New Diet Revolution

This popular, yet controversial, diet is based on the premise that people who are overweight are actually experiencing an overreaction of insulin to the carbohydrates that they eat. In people who have a large insulin response, blood glucose falls rapidly, causing hunger and resulting in overeating. To break this cycle, Atkins proposes a high-fat, low-carbohydrate diet, claiming that by increasing the fat in the diet, people will eat less because of the feeling of fullness that the fat can promote. However, carbohydrates are drastically restricted in the hope that insulin levels will stabilize and hunger will be suppressed. The additional benefit is that, since the brain needs glucose to survive, if it does not get what it needs from carbohydrates in the diet, the body will begin to break down fat cells as an alternate energy source.

Fallacy: There is no scientific proof that high insulin levels cause weight gain. There is, however, scientific proof that a diet high in saturated fats will increase the risk of heart disease and some forms of cancer. As the body burns its own fat reservoirs to make up for what is lacking in the diet, high levels of needed electrolytes such as calcium, potassium and sodium are lost in the urine. Because these are not being replaced in the diet, many potential problems are the result, including cardiac arrhythmia, osteoporosis, nausea, light-headedness and fatigue.

Many people claim to have lost weight on Dr. Atkins' diet plan, and that may be true, but it is a weight loss primarily due to a rapid loss of body fluids (needed to excrete the waste created from burning the body's own fat resources). This one premise can cause a host of other health concerns, including kidney problems.

The Ornish diet

Dr. Dean Ornish designed his diet plan to help patients reduce their risk of heart disease through full-sweeping lifestyle changes. His diet is a low-fat one, with reduced protein, but increased consumption of whole foods, fruits, vegetables, grains, beans and soy products. The Ornish diet has the most scientific support for its success in promoting weight loss. The main problem with it is gaining compliance. Its extreme limitations on fat often prove too difficult for any but the most dedicated and disciplined dieter to follow.

The zone diet

The zone diet is better known as the 30/30/40 diet, in which 30 percent of daily calories come from fat, 30 percent from protein and 40 percent from carbohydrates. These percentages were calculated to be the "optimal" ratio to control something called "eicosanoids," hormone-like compounds in the body thought to be involved in inflammation and certain diseases. It remains an open question as to whether this diet has any effect on eicosanoids or any disease process, but what is certain is that it restricts many foods in the fruits and vegetables category, which are known for their beneficial effects on health.

Sugar busters

The sugar buster diet proclaims, predictably, that all sugar is toxic to the human body. Therefore, foods that are high on the glycemic index are eliminated, and other foods low on the scale, such as whole grains, vegetables, fruits, lean meat and fiber, are consumed instead. The problem with this diet is that while it is reducing a person's sugar intake, other nutritious foods are eliminated, such as carrots, beets and potatoes. If you decide to follow this diet, chances are that you will lose weight, but you will open yourself up to greater health risks due to lacking nutrients. As with the Ornish diet, many people who begin the sugar busters diet start strong, but they cannot maintain it for any length of time due to its rigidity.

Most of the new fad diets that are on the market today are actually harmful to a person's health. They tend to run to one extreme or the other, containing excessive amounts of cholesterol, saturated fat or animal protein. They also tend to be lacking in many key nutrients necessary to counter disease. Other potential dangerous effects that have been noted include:

- Mild dehydration
- Headaches
- Nausea
- Sleep problems
- Fatigue
- Increased risk of osteoporosis
- Inability to maintain weight loss
- High blood pressure

Freedom From Fad Diets

So what is a person to do? I have good news: Through the combination of eating the right foods, burning calories through physical exercise and supplementing the diet with the proper nutrients, it is possible to lose the weight and keep it off! And not only can you do it without any detrimental effects to your body, but your health also will actually improve as a result of the changes that you make.

Foods that increase metabolism

As scientists continue to study the chemistry of the human body, five common groups of foods have been proven to increase metabolism and block the fatty acid uptake in the body's cells, thus causing a person to lose weight.

1. *Oatmeal.* The fiber found in common oatmeal has an incredible impact on the insulin levels in the bloodstream. When you eat sugary foods, the insulin converts those carbohydrates into fat storage and slows down your metabolism. But the fiber present in oatmeal blunts that insulin response. Anyone who is struggling to lose weight should fix themselves a bowl of oatmeal, or another type of oat bran cereal that is high in fiber, for breakfast. Fiber supplements such as apple pulp concentrate, citrus pectin and glucomannan, from the konjac plant, can also have the same effect.

2. *Salsa.* Spicy foods such as salsa, jalapeno peppers and cayenne peppers have been shown to increase the body's metabolism and burn more calories, even when the body is at rest. The chemical capsaicin, which actually causes the spiciness, is the key. One study showed that a single spicy meal increased people's metabolism by 25 percent, and the effect lasted for three hours.[2] I mention salsa in particular because the tomatoes contain lycopene, another helpful component in the prevention of breast cancer and prostate cancer.

3. *Green tea.* Certain chemicals within the green teas commonly found in Asian countries have been shown to increase the body's metabolic rate and increase the

breakdown and elimination of fat. The polyphenols present in the tea have a *thermogenic effect* on the body; that is, it causes the body to begin to burn its fat reservoirs. The amount of caffeine that is present in green tea, unlike the amount found in coffee, doesn't cause the jitters, but it does increase metabolism and allows the body to burn more calories while resting.

4. *Protein.* Diets that restrict protein intake are missing one important fact: Protein requires more calories to digest in the body than do carbohydrates or fats. To a certain extent, shifting to a higher protein diet will burn more calories and cause you to lose more weight. It is important not to go to an extreme with this, however, because too much protein can be harmful to the kidneys. It is also better to obtain protein in your diet from low-fat sources such as poultry and fish rather than from red meats.

5. *Fish.* The omega-3 fatty acids present in fish such as salmon, trout, mackerel, cod and sardines have consistently been shown to increase body metabolism.

Increased body metabolism is important because it increases the rate at which the body can burn fat while at rest. In other words, you can be "working off" those calories just by sitting in your chair! In fact, 65 to 70 percent of the total calories that you burn are burned while at rest, just to keep the heart beating, your intestines working, your food being digested in your system and other "automatic" processes. However, if you hope to lose weight and maintain good health, burning metabolic calories alone is not enough. Physical activity should be an important factor in any weight loss plan.

Burning calories through exercise

Different types of physical exercise will burn more or less calories, depending on the effort that is exerted. When I get out and run a seven-minute mile, I burn about 984 calories per hour. Walking at a moderate pace will burn about 246 calories per hour.

My wife, Linda, burns a lot of calories just working around the house. When she has to climb up and down the ladder to install the rain gutters around the house, she is burning 422 calories an hour. When she washes my car, if she does it vigorously enough, she burns 316 calories an hour.

And hanging the storm windows causes her to burn 352 calories an hour! Now, of course, I don't make my wife do those things, but my point is this: Make exercise a part of your life. Begin to take the stairs rather than the elevator. Park a little farther away from your destination and give yourself the opportunity for a brisk walk. And find a physical activity that suits you that you can stick to regularly.

Did you know that even working at the office can burn calories? Just by sitting at your desk doing paperwork, you burn 127 calories an hour. Taking a nap (sleeping) burns 63 calories an hour, but by far the most strenuous exercise, for those of you who are ready to snap yourself into shape, is cross-country skiing, uphill, which burns 1,160 calories per hour!

Physical activities that will help you control your weight will be the ones that you enjoy and will turn to on a consistent basis.

Natural supplements that promote weight loss

Many people who need to lose weight are intimidated by having to make sudden lifestyle changes such as changing their diets or starting up an intensive exercise program. Because of this, I encourage many of my patients to start simply, to do something they know they can do, such as taking supplements, indigenous to the natural plant kingdom, that will have a weight loss effect.

5-HTP (*Griffonia*)

5-HTP is a naturally occurring chemical found in *Griffonia*, a plant that is native to India. This chemical works differently from other weight loss products in that in the human body it is converted into the neurotransmitter serotonin. Serotonin, as we discussed earlier, has been found to be helpful for people facing memory problems, depression and anxiety. Lower doses of it will directly work on the hypothalamus gland within the brain, the gland that is responsible for the appetite.

Have you ever noticed that when you receive bad news over the phone, your appetite is suddenly gone? Your sudden change in mood has affected the serotonin levels in your brain, which in turn has affected your appetite center. So the benefit of 5-HTP is that it can control the food cravings that many overweight people experience, without side effects.

The urge to eat is built within human beings for the purpose of survival. Though it was created by God for a good purpose, in our fallen world, often God's good plans are twisted and distorted. What was once a healthy appetite gets out of control, and the deep, almost visceral cravings can get out of hand. If you feel that your food cravings are biological, you are right!

But thank God, He has provided a way out of every temptation, and in this case, it is through the 5-HTP He has provided in His plant kingdom. A dose of 100 milligrams is a sufficient dose for the purpose of weight loss.

Garcinia (hydroxycitric acid)

A second supplement from the plant kingdom comes from a gourd called a *garcinia,* which looks like a cross between an acorn squash and an orange. It contains the chemical *hydroxycitric acid,* which blocks the conversion of carbohydrates into fat storage. So, if you eat too many carbohydrates and they are not burned off as energy, they are not stored as fat as they usually would be. Instead, it turns those carbohydrates into glycogen, a harmless chemical that does not accumulate as fat. You should take a dose of 900 milligrams per day to help you lose weight.

Platycodon

One prescription that is often given by doctors to patients who need to lose weight is Xenical, a drug that decreases fat absorption in the body, but it is often accompanied by side effects such as diarrhea and other problems in the gastrointestinal tract. However, for centuries the plant *platycodon* has existed in China, which is now proving to have the same positive results in fat absorption and weight loss as Xenical, but with none of the negative side effects. Platycodon works by inhibiting the enzyme lipase, which causes the fat to be absorbed. A dose of 100 milligrams of the platycodon root is sufficient for weight loss.

Weight Loss Is Possible!

In conclusion, it is a myth that it is impossible to succeed at weight loss! The National Weight Control Registry began a study in the early 1990s that examined over three thousand people who were able to lose at least thirty pounds, and an average of sixty-six pounds, *and they kept it off for at least five and one-half years!*[3] Their pathway to successful weight loss was through changes in their diets and exercise patterns.

You can succeed despite your genetic profile! Seventy percent of the people involved in this study had at least one parent who was significantly overweight.

You can succeed despite your cravings! The people in this study didn't give up sweets altogether—they just drastically limited their intake. One person just ate the icing off of a cupcake and threw the rest of it away. Another person divided ice cream into tiny cubes and just ate one cube a day.

You can succeed without taking harmful "diet drugs" such as ephedra or fen-phen! These people modified their lifestyles rather than sending their bodies on a roller-coaster ride of highs and lows that many of the diet drugs cause.

You can succeed by finding God's pathway to healing (and weight loss) designed *just for you!*

ASK DR. CHERRY

QUESTION: **Do flavored green teas have the same weight-loss effect as ordinary green tea?**

ANSWER: Because green tea is traditionally an Asian tea, it is largely unfermented and not always palatable to many Americans. It is perfectly fine to use some of the flavored green teas that have come on the market today; they will have the same effect.

QUESTION: **I've heard that chocolate can be good for you. Is this true?**

ANSWER: Dark chocolate, without sugar, can be good for you due to the flavonoids it contains, which help to protect arteries.

QUESTION: **It is so hard to keep up a diet around Thanksgiving and Christmas. Do you have any suggestions for cooking around the holidays?**

ANSWER: The first suggestion that I have for people planning on eating big holiday dinners is to be careful not to exercise immediately afterwards. So many times, people will eat a big Thanksgiving meal that is full of fats and carbohydrates, and then that afternoon they try to go out and play a game of touch football with the kids, on a full stomach! That's a recipe for disaster; many heart attacks are caused by that scenario. So, if you must indulge in a big meal, take it easy on your body afterwards!

Of course, the best idea would be to cut down on the fat intake at those holiday dinners. Because it usually doesn't work to force yourself to forgo all of the goodies completely, there's usually a better chance fo success by making the food that you do eat healthier. Some ways to cut back on the fat include cooking the turkey with the skin on to keep in the flavor, but removing the skin before eating, because that is where most of the fat will be. Also, don't cook the stuffing inside of the turkey because it will absorb much of the fatty juices of the bird. And of course, watch the fat content of the gravy that you prepare; it doesn't do any good to eat the lean portions of the bird if you slather it with gravy that has twice as much fat!

My final suggestion has to do with the preparation of your meals. Be sure not to let food set out on the table too long before you put it back into the refrigerator; harmful bacteria don't take long to grow. Also, clean the cutting boards and other counter surfaces frequently with an antibacterial soap to avoid cross-contamination from salmonella or other bacteria that might be in uncooked meat or other foods.

Holidays such as Thanksgiving and Christmas are meant to be enjoyed! You can savor a delicious meal without completely sabotaging your diet by eating in moderation and not overindulging.

QUESTION: **I'm already taking Prozac for depression. Is it safe for me to take 5-HTP to try to lose some weight as well?**

ANSWER: No, it is not safe. If you are taking any type of antidepressant that changes the serotonin levels in your brain, such as Prozac, Zoloft or Celexa, you should not begin any 5-HTP treatments for weight loss, as you do not want to create too great of an effect. If you need to lose weight, try some of the other supplements or food suggestions listed in this chapter, or see your doctor for further instructions.

ESSENTIAL NUTRIENTS TO
ACHIEVE YOUR OPTIMAL WEIGHT

NATURAL SUBSTANCE	EFFECT	DAILY DOSAGE
Garcinia	Plant extract that helps suppress appetite and may help block the synthesis of fat in the body	900 mg
Glucomannan	Soluble fiber that slows the absorption of sugars from the intestinal tract, improves blood lipid levels and helps control appetite	1,500 mg
Absorbalean	Proprietary blend of natural fibers and herbs that helps regulate blood sugar and lipid levels	1,500 mg
Inulin	Plant extract with fiber-like qualities that enhances the growth of beneficial intestinal flora	800 mg
Green tea leaf	Herb with important antioxidant activity and phytochemicals that have been shown to increase the burning of fat for energy	200 mg
5-HTP	Amino acid derivative naturally found in the body that helps elevate mood and suppress the appetite	100 mg
Platycodon root	Herb traditionally used in China and other Asian countries to prevent obesity	100 mg
Cayenne pepper	Herb with thermogenic properties and natural appetite-suppressing activity	10 mg

SECTION THREE

APPENDICES

RECOMMENDED DOSES FOR BASIC NUTRIENT SUPPORT

NUTRIENT	SUPPORT FUNCTION	DAILY DOSAGE
Biotin	Essential vitamin for healthy skin, hair and nails	300 mcg
Carotenoid complex	Important group of phytonutrients with antioxidant activity	2,000 mcg
Folic acid	Essential vitamin needed for normal growth and development	600 mcg
Vitamin A (beta carotene; retinyl palmitate)	Essential vitamin important for the eyes, skin, bones, immune and reproductive systems	25,000 IU
Vitamin B$_1$ (thiamin)	Essential vitamin needed for energy metabolism	50 mg
Vitamin B$_2$ (riboflavin)	Essential vitamin needed for energy metabolism	50 mg
Vitamin B$_3$ (niacin/ niacinamide)	Essential vitamin needed for energy metabolism	100 mg
Vitamin B$_5$ (calcium pantothenate)	Essential vitamin needed in energy production pathways	50 mg
Vitamin B$_6$ (pyridoxine)	Essential vitamin needed for amino acid metabolism, neurotransmitter synthesis, glycogen utilization, immune function and homocysteine regulation	75 mg
Vitamin B$_{12}$	Essential vitamin needed for proper blood cell formation and cell division	100 mcg
Vitamin C	Essential vitamin needed for its antioxidant activities and for connective tissue repair and regeneration	2,000 mg

NUTRIENT	SUPPORT FUNCTION	DAILY DOSAGE
Vitamin D₃ (cholecalciferol)	Essential vitamin needed for proper calcium metabolism	400 IU
Vitamin E (d-alpha toco-pheryl succinate)	Natural, stabilized form of vitamin E that protects cells from free-radical damage	800 IU
Boron	Essential mineral that strengthens bones and supports joint health	2,000 mcg
Calcium	Essential mineral important for bones, teeth, muscles and nerves	1,000 mg
Chromium	Essential mineral that improves glucose metabolism	300 mcg
Copper	Essential mineral needed for connective tissue, immune function and nerve cells	2 mg
Hydromins	Natural source of trace minerals essential to life	50 mg
Iodine	Essential mineral needed for proper thyroid function	150 mcg
Magnesium	Essential mineral important for bones, nerves, heart and muscles	400 mg
Manganese	Essential mineral with antioxidant and connective tissue functions	7.5 mg
Molybdenum	Essential mineral important to many key metabolic pathways	75 mcg
Potassium	Essential mineral important for fluid balance and nerve cell conduction	99 mg
Selenium	Essential mineral with antioxidant activity	200 mcg
Silica	Essential mineral important for skin, bones, cartilage and the immune system	7.5 mg
Vanadium	Trace mineral shown to support insulin function and glucose regulation	300 mcg

NUTRIENT	SUPPORT FUNCTION	DAILY DOSAGE
Zinc	Essential mineral important for skin, bones, cartilage, and the immune system	15 mg
Choline	Essential nutrient that aids in fat metabolism and supports memory function	250 mg
Inositol	Nutrient that supports the health and function of the nervous system	50 mg
Phosphatidylserine	Phospholipid nutrient that supports brain and nerve cell function	100 mcg
Fruits and greens powder	Concentrated source of phytonutrients from twenty-four fruits and vegetables	300 mg
Olive leaf extract	Herb that supports cardiovascular and immune function	20 mg
Bioperine	Enhances absorption of a wide range of nutrients	6 mg
Bromelain	Enzyme that aids in protein digestion	50 mg
Cinnamon powder	Herb traditionally used as an aid to digestion	80 mg
Fennel seed powder	Herb traditionally used to support and enhance digestion	80 mg
Glucono-delta-lactone	Promotes healthy growth of beneficial microflora in the intestines	300 mg
Multi-enzyme complex	Mixture of enzymes that aid in the digestion of carbohydrates, fats and proteins	50 mg
Papain	Enzyme from papaya that helps with protein digestion	25 mg
Peppermint leaf powder	Herb traditionally used to improve digestion	80 mg

NUTRIENT	SUPPORT FUNCTION	DAILY DOSAGE
Glucomannan	Soluble fiber that helps curb appetite, regulate blood sugar and promote cholesterol excretion	150 mg
Alpha lipoic acid	Unique antioxidant and co-factor for energy production	50 mg
Bilberry fruit powder	Natural source of flavonoid and anthocyanidin antioxidants	25 mg
Broccoli powder	Natural source of antioxidants and beneficial phytochemicals	50 mg
Cabbage powder	Natural source of antioxidants and beneficial phytochemicals	50 mg
Citrus bioflavonoids	Important group of phytonutrients that enhance the activity of vitamin C	150 mg
Coenzyme Q_{10}	Nutrient essential to energy production in the heart and muscles	25 mg
Glutathione	Important antioxidant and detoxifier in the body	10 mg
Grape seed extract	Natural source of powerful polyphenolic antioxidants	50 mg
Grape skin extract	Natural source of powerful polyphenolic antioxidants	25 mg
Green tea extract	Natural source of catechin antioxidants	50 mg
Lycopene	Carotenoid antioxidant essential for proper functioning of the prostate	1,000 mcg
N-acetyl-L-cysteine	Important antioxidant and detoxifier in the body	50 mg
PABA (para-amino benzoic acid)	Nutrient that supports proper cell growth and development	10 mg

NUTRIENT	SUPPORT FUNCTION	DAILY DOSAGE
Quercetin	Flavonoid antioxidant with anti-inflammatory and antihistamine activity	25 mg
Rutin	Flavonoid antioxidant that supports the strength and integrity of blood vessels	25 mg
Tocotrienol complex	Part of the vitamin E complex with important antioxidant and cholesterol-regulating activity	5 mg
Tomato powder	Natural source of lycopene and other carotenoids	50 mg
Vitamin E (mixed tocopherols)	Part of the vitamin E complex with important antioxidant activity	5 IU
Evening primrose oil	Source of essential fatty acids that support the skin, joints and immune system	1,000 mg
Marine oils	Natural source of heart-healthy essential fatty acids	2,000 mg

Appendix B

Recipes for Healthy Living

Cancer-Fighting Lentil Soup

4 Tbsp. extra-virgin olive oil
2 boneless, skinless chicken breasts, all visible fat removed, cubed
12.3-oz. carton firm tofu, cut in cubes
2 stalks celery, chopped
¾ cup shiitake mushrooms, chopped
2 cloves garlic, chopped
1 leek, trimmed of root and green top, chopped
½ cup onion, chopped
½ cup fresh parsley, chopped
½ cup baby carrots, cut in small slices
2.25 oz. sliced black olives, drained
¼ tsp. ground ginger
¼–½ tsp. pure ginseng powder*, to taste
2 14-oz. cans, low-sodium, fat-free chicken broth
3 14-oz. cans of water
1 pound bag lentils, sorted and rinsed

In large soup pot, sauté chicken and tofu in olive oil until chicken is white. Remove both from oil and set aside.

Sauté celery, mushrooms, garlic, leek, onion, parsley and carrots until vegetables are crisp tender. Add black olives, ginger, ginseng, chicken broth and water. Return chicken and tofu to vegetable mixture. Add lentils. Stir well.

Cook on medium-high heat for 60 minutes or until lentils are tender. Stir occasionally.

* NOTE: It is important to use American ginseng (Panax quinquefolium). You can search for company names such as CSI Ginseng Products and Pacific Rim Ginseng. Ginseng has an "earthy" and bitter taste; therefore, it is wise to start with small amounts in cooking and taste-test for desired amounts.

Breadcrumb-Coated Chicken Breasts

1 cup orange juice
1 Tbsp. minced garlic
2 Tbsp. low-sodium soy sauce
1 tsp. olive oil
4–6 boneless, skinless chicken breasts, trimmed of any fat
1 cup whole-wheat breadcrumbs
2 tsp. dried basil, crushed
2 tsp. paprika
¼ tsp. ground red pepper
¼ tsp. ground black pepper

In 9" x 13" nonmetal dish, mix orange juice, garlic, soy sauce and olive oil. Pierce both sides of chicken breasts with fork. Place chicken in mixture and turn to coat both sides well. Cover and refrigerate for 1 hour.

Preheat oven to 350° F. Coat large baking sheet with no-cholesterol cooking spray.

In shallow bowl, mix breadcrumbs, basil, paprika, red pepper and black pepper.

Drain marinade from chicken and discard. Coat chicken well on both sides with breadcrumb mixture. Place on baking sheet. Bake for 20–30 minutes or until chicken is no longer pink in center when tested with sharp knife.

Spinach With Apples and Walnuts— a Favorite in France

8 cups fresh spinach, well rinsed
3 Tbsp. extra-virgin olive oil
½ small onion, finely chopped
2 medium to large red delicious apples, peeled, cored and diced
6 Tbsp. chopped walnuts
Lite salt and pepper to taste

Place dripping wet spinach in large pot covered with lid. Cook over high heat for about 3 minutes or until spinach is reduced in volume and slightly softened. Shake pot frequently while cooking without lifting lid. Drain well, and press liquid from spinach.

Heat olive oil in large skillet. Sauté onion and apples until onion has softened. (Do not "brown" onion.) Stir in walnuts, and continue cooking for 5 minutes. Add spinach, and sauté for 3 minutes longer.

Season with Lite salt and pepper. Serve immediately.

Zucchini Pie

2 large eggs, slightly beaten
¼ cup extra-virgin olive oil
¼ tsp. rubbed sage
½ tsp. Lite salt
¼ tsp. ground black pepper
¾ cup biscuit mix
¾ cup cheddar cheese, 2 percent fat, shredded
1 small onion, chopped
2 cups zucchini, shredded

Prepare 9-inch glass pie pan with no-cholesterol cooking spray.

In large mixing bowl, slightly beat eggs; then add remaining ingredients in order, stirring to blend well. Pour mixture into pie pan. Bake at 350° F for 45 minutes.

Cool for 10 minutes. Slice in pie wedges. Serve with fresh green salad with cherry tomatoes and your favorite fat-free salad dressing.

Good on a cold winter night!

New Potatoes and Green Beans With Pesto

4 cups small new potatoes, washed and cut in half
4 cups fresh green beans, washed and trimmed

Pesto ingredients:
2 Tbsp. chopped walnuts
1 garlic clove, peeled
3 Tbsp. fresh basil leaves
6 Tbsp. freshly grated low-fat Parmesan cheese
5 Tbsp. extra-virgin olive oil
¼ tsp. Lite salt
Pinch of black pepper

Boil potatoes for about 10 minutes or until tender.
Boil green beans for about 5 minutes or until tender.

Place remaining ingredients in food processor. Process only until the basil is well chopped (about 10 seconds).

Drain potatoes and green beans. Toss with pesto and serve.

Polenta Casserole

2 tsp. olive oil, divided
2 cups onion, chopped
3 cups (12 oz.) mushrooms, coarsely chopped
1½ tsp. Lite salt, divided
2 cloves garlic, chopped
½ cup dry red wine
1 tsp. dried rosemary (or 1 Tbsp. fresh, chopped)
1 Tbsp. tomato paste
1 can (14½-oz.) diced tomatoes, undrained
4 cups water
1 cup instant polenta (i.e., Contadina brand)
1 cup fresh grated Parmesan cheese
¼ tsp. black pepper, divided
½ cup part-skim ricotta cheese
1½ tsp. olive oil (for top layer)

Preheat oven to 400° F.

Heat 1 teaspoon oil in 10-inch cast iron skillet over medium-high heat. Add onion; sauté for 8 minutes. Add mushrooms, ½ teaspoon salt and garlic. Cook 4 minutes, stirring frequently. Stir in wine, rosemary and tomato paste. Reduce heat to medium. Cook 3 minutes. Stir in tomatoes, and cook about 10 minutes until thick. Remove from heat.

Bring water to a boil in saucepan. Stir in polenta and remaining 1 teaspoon salt. Reduce heat to low. Cook until thick (about 5 minutes), stirring frequently.

Spread ⅓ of polenta mixture into 9" x 13" baking dish coated with 1 teaspoon oil. Spread half of tomato sauce mixture over polenta. Top with 2 tablespoons Parmesan cheese and ⅛ teaspoon pepper. Drop half of the ricotta cheese by spoonfuls onto Parmesan cheese. Repeat layers, ending with polenta. Top with ¼ cup Parmesan cheese and drizzle with 1½ teaspoons olive oil.

Bake at 400° for 25 minutes or until bubbly. Serves 6.

I love this Mediterranean dish, and I hope you do, too!

NATURAL FOODS TO PEP YOU UP!

- Whole-grain bread, especially those with added nuts and seeds

- Whole-grain cereals, brown rice, pearl barley and oat cakes

- Root vegetables like carrots, turnips and potatoes

- Cruciferous plants like broccoli and cauliflower

- Legumes like lentils, kidney beans and soybeans

- Fresh fruits like bananas, melon, plums, grapes and oranges

- Ready-to-eat dried apricots, dates, figs and prunes

- Oily fish like salmon and tuna

- Nuts, especially almonds and seeds

HEALING
SCRIPTURES

Don't be impressed with your own wisdom. Instead, fear the LORD and turn your back on evil. Then you will gain renewed health and vitality.

—PROVERBS 3:7–8, NLT

If thou wilt diligently hearken to the voice of the LORD thy God, and wilt do that which is right in his sight, and wilt give ear to his commandments, and keep all his statutes, I will put none of these diseases upon thee, which I have brought upon the Egyptians: for I am the LORD that healeth thee.

—EXODUS 15:26

Worship the LORD your God, and his blessing will be on your food and water. I will take away sickness from among you, and none will miscarry or be barren in your land. I will give you a full life span.

—EXODUS 23:25–26, NIV

And he stood over her, and rebuked the fever; and it left her: and immediately she arose and ministered unto them.

—LUKE 4:39

Now when the sun was setting, all they that had any sick with divers diseases brought them unto him; and he laid his hands on every one of them, and healed them.

—LUKE 4:40

And looking round about upon them all, he said unto the man, Stretch forth thy hand. And he did so: and his hand was restored whole as the other.

—LUKE 6:10

As he went along, he saw a man blind from birth…he spit on the ground, made some mud with the saliva, and put it on the man's eyes. "Go," he told him, "wash in the Pool of Siloam" (this word means Sent). So the man went and washed, and came home seeing.

—JOHN 9:1, 6–7, NIV

Then God said, "I give you every seed-bearing plant on the face of the whole earth and every tree that has fruit with seed in it. They will be yours for food."

—GENESIS 1:29, NIV

There will be mighty and violent earthquakes, and in various places famines and pestilences (plagues: malignant and contagious or infectious epidemic diseases which are deadly and devastating); and there will be sights of terror and great signs from heaven.

—LUKE 21:11, AMP

But he was wounded for our transgressions, he was bruised for our iniquities: the chastisement of our peace was upon him; and with his stripes we are healed.

—ISAIAH 53:5

Who his own self bare our sins in his own body on the tree, that we, being dead to sins, should live unto righteousness: by whose stripes ye were healed.

—1 PETER 2:24

I will praise thee; for I am fearfully and wonderfully made.

—PSALM 139:14

Be strong and let your heart take courage, all you who wait for and hope for and expect the Lord!

—PSALM 31:24, AMP

Peace I leave with you, My peace I give to you; not as the world gives do I give to you. Let not your heart be troubled, neither let it be afraid.

—JOHN 14:27, NKJV

The thief cometh not, but for to steal, and to kill, and to destroy: I am come that they might have life, and that they might have it more abundantly.

—JOHN 10:10

He who does not use his endeavors to heal himself is brother to him who commits suicide.

—PROVERBS 18:9, AMP

Casting all your care upon him, for he careth for you.

—1 PETER 5:7

The leaves of the tree were for the healing of the nations.

—REVELATION 22:2, NKJV

The effective, fervent prayer of a righteous man avails much.

—JAMES 5:16, NKJV

The LORD will keep you free from every disease.

—DEUTERONOMY 7:15, NIV

He sent His word and healed them.

—PSALM 107:20, NKJV

"But I will restore you to health and heal your wounds," declares the LORD.

—JEREMIAH 30:17, NIV

They will place their hands on sick people, and they will get well.

—MARK 16:18, NIV

Pray without ceasing.

—1 THESSALONIANS 5:17

Praying always with all prayer and supplication in the Spirit, and watching thereunto with all perseverance.

—EPHESIANS 6:18

My son, do not forget my law, but let your heart keep my commands; for length of days and long life and peace they will add to you.

—PROVERBS 3:1–2, NKJV

He will redeem their life from oppression and violence; and precious shall be their blood in His sight.

—PSALM 72:14, NKJV

Heal me, O LORD, and I shall be healed; save me, and I shall be saved, for You are my praise.

—JEREMIAH 17:14, NKJV

"Because he loves me," says the LORD, "I will rescue him; I will protect him, for he acknowledges my name. He will call upon me, and I will answer him; I will be with him in trouble, I will deliver him and honor him. With long life will I satisfy him and show him my salvation."

—PSALM 91:14–16, NIV

Thus says the LORD, the God of David your father: "I have heard your prayer, I have seen your tears; surely I will heal you."

—2 KINGS 20:5, NKJV

And Jesus went about all Galilee, teaching in their synagogues, and preaching the gospel of the kingdom, and healing all manner of sickness and all manner of disease among the people.

—MATTHEW 4:23

Great multitudes followed him, and he healed them all.

—MATTHEW 12:15

Be not wise in your own eyes; reverently fear and worship the Lord and turn [entirely] away from evil. It shall be health to your nerves and sinews, and marrow and moistening to your bones.

—PROVERBS 3:7–8, AMP

Then your light shall break forth like the morning, your healing shall spring forth speedily.

—ISAIAH 58:8, NKJV

He heals the brokenhearted and binds up their wounds.

—PSALM 147:3, NIV

Bless the LORD, O my soul: and all that is within me, bless his holy name. Bless the LORD, O my soul, and forget not all his benefits: Who forgiveth all thine iniquities; who healeth all thy diseases.

—PSALM 103:1–3

Moses was 120 years old when he died, yet his eyesight was perfect and he was as strong as a young man.

—DEUTERONOMY 34:7, TLB

Pay attention, my child, to what I say. Listen carefully. Don't lose sight of my words. Let them penetrate deep within your heart, for they bring life and radiant health to anyone who discovers their meaning…Look straight ahead, and fix your eyes on what lies

before you. Mark out a straight path for your feet; then stick to the path and stay safe.
—PROVERBS 4:20–22, 25–26, NLT

I will lift up my eyes to the hills—from whence comes my help?
—PSALM 121:1, NKJV

As the sun went down that evening, all the villagers who had any sick people in their homes, no matter what their diseases were, brought them to Jesus; and the touch of his hands healed every one!
—LUKE 4:40, TLB

Now a woman, having a flow of blood for twelve years, who had spent all of her livelihood on physicians and could not be healed by any, came from behind and touched the border of His garment. And immediately her flow of blood stopped.
—LUKE 8:43–44, NKJV

He personally carried away our sins in his own body on the cross so we can be dead to sin and live for what is right. You have been healed by his wounds!
—1 PETER 2:24, NLT

For God has not given us a spirit of fear, but of power and of love and of a sound mind.
—2 TIMOTHY 1:7, NKJV

Bless the LORD, O my soul, and forget not all His benefits… Who satisfies your mouth with good things, so that your youth is renewed like the eagle's.
—PSALM 103:2, 5, NKJV

Chapter 5
Beating Heart Disease

1. American Heart Association, *Heart Disease and Stroke Statistics—2003 Update* (Dallas, TX: American Heart Association, 2002).

2. J. R. Berrazueta et al., "The Incidence of Arrhythmias in Young Persons Without Demonstrable Heart Disease: A 24-Hour Holter Study in 100 Medical Students," *Rev Esp Cardiol* 46(3) (March 1993): 146–151.

3. F. Lopez-Jimenez, "Heavy Meals May Trigger Heart Attacks," American Heart Association Scientific Sessions 2000, November 12–15, 2000, New Orleans.

4. U. Schmidt et al., "Efficacy of Hawthorn Preparation LI132 in 78 Patients With Chronic Congestive Heart Failure Defined As NYHA Functional Class II," *Phytomed.* (1994): 1:17–24.

5. L. Alcocer et al., "A Comparative Study of Policosanol Versus Acipimox in Patients With Type II Hypercholesterolemia," *Int. J. Tissue React.* 21 (1999): 85–92.

Chapter 6
Lower High Blood Pressure—Naturally

1. L. A. Ferrara et al., "Olive Oil and Reduced Need for Antihypertensive Medications," *Archives of Internal Medicine* 160(6) (May 27, 2000): 837–842.

2. Ibid.

3. J. C. Witterman et al., "A Prospective Study of Nutritional Factors and Hypertension Among U.S. Women," *Circulation* 80(5) (November 1989): 1320–1327. A. Ascherio et al., "A Prospective Study of Nutritional Factors and Hypertension Among U.S. Men," *Circulation* 86(5) (November 1992): 1475–1484.

4. M. R. Joffres, D. M. Reed and K. Yano, "Relationship of Magnesium Intake and Other Dietary Factors to Blood Pressure: the Honolulu Heart Study," *Am J Clin Nutr* 45(2) (February 1987): 469–476.

5. American Heart Association, *Heart Disease and Stroke Statistics—2003 Update.*

6. Y. Kawano et al., "Effects of Magnesium Supplementation in Hypertensive Patients," *Hypertension* 32 (1998): 260–265. J. C. Witteman et al., "Reduction of Blood Pressure With Oral Magnesium Supplementation in Women With Mild to Moderate Hypertension," *Am J Clin Nutr* 60 (July 1994): 129–135. T. Motoyama et al., "Oral Magnesium Supplementation in Patients With Essential Hypertension," *Hypertension* 13 (1989): 227–232.

7. N. M. Rao et al., "Angiotensin Converting Enzyme Inhibitors From Ripened and Unripened Bananas," *Curr Sci* 76 (1999): 86–88.

Chapter 7
Prevent Hardening of the Arteries

1. American Heart Association, *Heart Disease and Stroke Statistics—2003 Update.*

Chapter 8
Balancing the Immune System

1. L. C. Clark et al., "Effects of Selenium Supplementation for Cancer Prevention in Patients With Carcinoma of the Skin: A Randomized Controlled Trial, Nutritional Prevention of Cancer Study Group" [published erratum appears in *JAMA* 277 (19) (May 21, 1997): 1520], *JAMA* 276 (1996): 1957–1963.

2. E. Lansky et al., "Further Studies on Pomegranate and Breast Cancer," presented at the IV Madrid Breast Cancer Conference, June 7–9, 2001, Madrid, Spain.

3. Z. Zakay-Ranes et al., "Inhibition of Several Strains of Influenza Virus In Vitro and Reduction of Symptoms by an Elderberry Extract (Sambucus nigra L.) During an Outbreak of Influenza B. Panama," *J Altern. Med.* 1 (1995): 361–369.

4. A. T. Borchers et al., "Mushrooms, Tumors, and Immunity," *Proc Soc Exp Biol Med* 221(4) (1999): 281–293.

Chapter 9
Protect Yourself From Colds and Flu

1. M. Takahashi and T. Yamada, "Influenza A Virus and Parkinson's Disease," *Neurosci News* 2(3–4) (1999): 93–101.

Chapter 10
Diabetes: Starving in the Land of Plenty

1. Centers for Disease Control and Prevention, "National Diabetes Fact Sheet: General Information and National Estimates on Diabetes in

the United States, 2000" (Atlanta, GA: U.S. Department of Health and Human Services, Centers for Disease Control and Prevention, 2002).

2. Ibid.

3. K. A. Meyer et al., "Carbohydrates, Dietary Fiber, and Incident Type 2 Diabetes in Older Women," *Am J Clin Nutr* 72 (2000): 921–930.

4. J. Anderson et al., "Effects of Psyllium on Glucose and Serum Lipid Responses in Men With Type 2 Diabetes and Hypocholesterolemia," *Am J Clin Nutr* 70 (1999): 466–473.

5. L. Ali et al., "Studies on Hypoglycemic Effects of Fruit Pulp, Seed, and Whole Plant of Momordica Charantia on Normal and Diabetic Model Rats," *Planta Med* 59 (1993): 408–412. C. Day et al., "Hypoglycaemic Effect of Momordica Charantia Extracts," *Planta Med* 56 (1990): 426–429. B. A. Leatherdale et al., "Improvement in Glucose Tolerance Due to Momordica Charantia (Karela)," *Br Med J (Clin Res Ed)* 282(6279) (1981): 1823–1824. A. Raman and C. Lau, "Anti-Diabetic Properties and Phytochemistry of *Momordica Charantia* L (Curcurbitaceae)," *Phytomed Res* 2 (1996): 349–362.

6. S. J. Persaud et al., "Gymnema Sylvestre Stiumlates Insulin Release In Vitro by Increased Membrane Permeability," *J. Endocrinol.* 163(2) (1999): 207–212. E. R. Shanmugasundaram et al., "Use of Gynmena Sylvestre Leaf Extract in the Control of Blood Glucose in Insulin-Dependent Diabetes Mellitus," *J Ethnopharmacol.* 30(3) (1990): 281–294.

Chapter 13
Natural Relief for Irritable Bowel Syndrome

1. M. H. Pittler and E. Ernst, "Peppermint Oil for Irritable Bowel Syndrome: A Critical Review and Metaanalysis," *The American Journal of Gastroenterology* 93(7) (1998): 1131–1135. J. H. Liu et al., "Enteric-Coated Peppermint Oil Capsules in the Treatment of Irritable Bowel Syndrome: A Prospective, Randomized Trial," *Journal of Gastroenterology* 32 (1997): 765–768. M. J. Dew, B. K. Evans and J. Rhodes, "Peppermint Oil for the Irritable Bowel Syndrome: A Multicenter Trial," *Br J Clin Pract* 38 (1984): 394–398.

2. Dew, Evans and Rhodes, "Peppermint Oil for the Irritable Bowel Syndrome: A Multicenter Trial."

3. M. Camilleri, "Therapeutic Approach to the Patient With Irritable Bowel Syndrome," *The American Journal of Medicine* (5A) (1999). R. B. Lynn, "Current Concepts: Irritable Bowel Syndrome," *New England Journal of Medicine* 329 (1993). *Mayo Clinic Family Health Book* (n.p.:

William Morrow & Co., 1996). *Applied Therapeutics: The Clinical Use of Drugs* (n.p.: Applied Therapeutics, 1995). *Micromedex Healthcare Series* (n.p.: Micromedex, Inc., 2001). *Washington Manual of Medical Therapeutics* (n.p.: Lippincott-Raven Publishers, 1998). *Griffith's 5-Minute Clinical Consult* (n.p.: Lippincott, Williams & Wilkins, Inc., 1999). *Sleisenger & Fordtran's Gastrointestinal and Liver Disease* (n.p.: W. B. Saunders Company, 1998).

Chapter 14
Natural Solutions for Arthritis

1. "Arthritis Prevalence and Activity Limitations—United States 1990," *Morbidity and Mortality Weekly Report (MMWR)* 43 (1994): 433

2. H. Wang et al., "Antioxidant and Anti-Inflammatory Activities of Anthocyanins and Their Aglycone, Cyanidin, From Tart Cherries," *Journal of Natural Products* 62 (1999): 294–296.

3. V. K. Pachnanda et al., *Ind J Pharm* 13 (1981): 63.

4. H. P. Amman et al., "Mechanism of Anti-Inflammatory Actions of Curcumine and Boswellic Acids," *J Ethnopharmacol* 38 (1993): 113–119.

5. J. Y. Reginster et al., "Long-Term Effects of Glucosamine Sulfate on Osteoarthritis Progression: A Randomized, Placebo-Controlled Trial," *Lancet* 357 (2001): 251–256.

6. S. Taussig, "The Mechanism of the Physiological Action of Bromelain," *Medical Hypothesis* 6(1) (1980): 99–104.

7. J. L. Blonstein, "Control of Swelling in Boxing Injuries," *Practitioner* 203 (1969): 206.

8. G. Crolle and E. D'Este, "Glucosamine Sulphate for the Management of Arthrosis: A Controlled Clinical Investigation," *Curr Med Res Opin* 7 (1980): 104–109. J. C. Delafuente, "Glucosamine in the Treatment of Osteoarthritis," *Rheum Dis Clin North Am* 26 (1) (February 2000): 1–11, vii. G. S. Kelly, "The Role of Glucosamine Sulfate and Chondroitin Sulfates in the Treatment of Degenerative Joint Disease," *Altern. Med. Rev.* 3 (1998): 27–39. E. D'Ambrosio et al., "Glucosamine Sulphate: A Controlled Clinical Investigation in Arthrosis," *Pharmatherapeutica* 2(8) (1981): 504–508.

Chapter 15
Alzheimer's Disease and Other Memory Problems

1. Alzheimer's Association, "Facts About Alzheimer's Disease, 2002."

Chapter 16
Freedom From Depression and Anxiety

1. L. J. van Hiele, "1-5-Hydroxytryptophan in Depression: The First Substitution Therapy in Psychiatry? The Treatment of 99 Outpatients with 'Therapy-Resistant' Depressions," *Neuropsychobiology* 6(4) (1980): 230–240.

2. T. C. Birdsall, "5-Hydroxytryptophan: A Clinically Effective Serotonin Precursor," *Altern Med Rev* 3(4) (August 1998): 271–280. G. Bono et al., "L-5HTP Treatment in Primary Headaches: An Attempt at Clinical Identification of Responsive Patients," *Cephalalgia* 4(3) (September 1984): 159–165. G. De Giorgis et al., "Headache in Association With Sleep Disorders in Children: A Psychodiagnostic Evaluation and Controlled Clinical Study—L 5-HTP versus Placebo," *Drugs Exp Clin Res* 13 (1987): 425–433.

Chapter 17
Herbal Treatments for Headaches and Dizziness

1. A. Grontved et al., "Ginger Root Against Seasickness: A Controlled Trial on the Open Sea," *Acta Otolaryngol* 105 (1998): 45–49.

Chapter 18
Natural Remedies for Vision Problems

1. J. T. Landrum et al., "A One-Year Study of the Macular Pigment: The Effect of 140 Days of a Lutein Supplement," *Exp. Eye Res.* 65 (1997): 57–62.

Chapter 19
Natural Remedies for Prostate Enlargement

1. J. D. McConnell, "Epidemiology, Etiology, Pathophysiology, and Diagnosis of Benign Prostatic Hyperplasia," in P. C. Walsh et al., eds., *Campbell's Urology,* vol. 2, 7th edition (Philadelphia: W. B. Saunders Company, 1998), 1429–1452.

2. T. Wilt et al., "Pygeum Africanum for Benign Prostatic Hyperplasia," *Cochran Database Syst Rev* 1 (2002): CD001044. T. J. Wilt et al., "Phytotherapy for Benigh Prostatic Hyperplasia," *Public Health Nutr* 3(4A) (December 2000): 459–472. J. Breza et al., "Efficacy and Acceptability of Tadenan (Pygeum Africanum Extract) in the Treatment of Benign Prostatic Hyperplasia (BPH): A Multicentre Trial in Central Europe," *Curr Med Res Opin* 14(3) (1998): 127–139.

3. L. S. Marks et al., "Effects of a Saw Palmetto Herbal Blend in Men With Symptomatic Benign Prostatic Hyperplasia," *J Urol* 163(5) (May

2000): 1451–1456. G. S. Gerber, "Saw Palmetto for the Treatment of Men With Lower Urinary Tract Symptoms," *J Urol* 163(5) (May 2000): 1408–1412. A. Cristoni, F. Di Pierro and E. Bombardelli, "Botanical Derivatives for the Prostate," *Filoterapia* 71 Suppl 1 (August 2000): S21–S28. T. J. Wilt et al., "Saw Palmetto Extracts for Treatment of Benign Prostatic Hyperplasia: A Systematic Review," *JAMA* 280(18) (November 11, 1998): 1604–1609.

Chapter 20
Natural Remedies for Symptoms of Menopause

1. M. T. Goodman et al., "Association of Soy and Fiber Consumption With the Risk of Endometrial Cancer," *Am J Epidemiol* 146(4) (August 15, 1997): 294–306.
2. C. M. Hasler, "The Cardiovascular Effects of Soy Products," *J Cardiovasc Nurs* 16(4) (July 2002): 50–63. M. J. Messina, "Soy Foods and Soybean Isoflavones and Menopausal Health," *Nutr Clin Care* 5(6) (November–December 2002): 272–282. L. W. Lissin and J. P. Cooke, "Phytoestrogens and Coronary Heart Disease," *J Am Coll Cardiol* 35(6) (May 2000): 1403–1410. T. B. Clarkson and M. S. Anthony, "Phyoestrogens and Coronary Heart Disease," *Baillieres Clin Endocrinol Metab* 12(4) (December 1998): 589–604.

Chapter 21
PMS: Stopping the Monthly Plague

1. The American College of Obstetricians and Gynecologists, *Clinical Management Guidelines* no. 15 (April 2000).
2. C. Lauritzen et al., "Treatment of Premenstrual Tension Syndrome With Vitex Agnus Castus. Controlled, Double-Blind Study Versus Pyridoxine," *Phytomedicine* 4 (1997): 183–189.

Chapter 22
Reversing the Effects of Varicose Veins

1. T. E. Bielanski and Z. H. Piotrowski, "Horse Chestnut Seed Extract for Chronic Venous Insufficiency," *J Fam Pract.* 48(3) (March 1999): 171–172. H. Bisler et al., "[Effects of Horse Chestnut Seed Extract on Transcapillary Filtration in Chronic Venous Insufficiency]," *Dtsch Med Wochenschr.* 111(35) (August 29, 1986): 1321–1329.
2. U. Siebert et al., "Efficacy, Routine Effectiveness, and Safety of Horse Chestnut Seed Extract in the Treatment of Chronic Venous Insufficiency. A Meta-Analysis of Randomized Controlled Trials and Large Observational Studies," *Int Angiol* 21(4) (December 2002):

305–315. M. H. Pittler and E. Ernst, "Horse Chestnut Seed Extract for Chronic Venous Insufficiency. A Criteria-Based Systematic Review," *Arch Dermatol* 134(11) (November 1998): 1356–1360. C. Diehm et al., "Comparison of Leg Compression Stocking and Oral Horse Chestnut Seed Extract Therapy in Patients With Chronic Venous Insufficiency," *Lancet* 347(8997) (February 3, 1996): 292–294.

Chapter 24
The Fallacy of Fad Diets

1. Partnership for Healthy Weight Management, Body Mass Index, retrieved from the Internet at www.consumer.gov/weightloss/bmi.htm.

2. C. J. Henry and B. Emery, "Effect of Spiced Food on Metabolic Rate," *Hum Nutr Clin Nutr.* 40 (1986): 165–168.

3. M. L. Klem et al., "A Descriptive Study of Individuals Successful at Long-Term Maintenance of Substantial Weight Loss," *Amer J of Clinical Nutrition* 66 (1997): 239–246.

SELECTED REFERENCES

Thousands of references and scientific articles were reviewed for this book, and it is not possible to list them all. You will find listed, however, some of the most relevant and interesting scientific publications that are available at medical libraries. Much of the research was obtained by interviews with research scientists and experts in their fields. In addition, news reports from conferences, lectures, and scientific papers were used in the preparation of this book.

Adlercreutz, H., and W. Mazur. "Phyto-Estrogens and Western Diseases." *Ann Med* 29 (1997): 95–120.

Albanes, D., et al. "Alpha-Tocopherol and Beta-Carotene Supplements and Lung Cancer Incidence in the Alpha-Tocopherol, Beta-Carotene Cancer Prevention Study: Effects of Base-Line Characteristics and Study Compliance." *J Natl Cancer Inst* 88 (1996): 1560–1570.

Albert, C. M., et al. "Fish Consumption and Risk of Sudden Cardiac Death." *JAMA* 279 (1998): 23–28.

Albertazzi, P., et al. "The Effect of Dietary Soy Supplementation on Hot Flashes." *Obstet Gynecol* 91 (1998): 6–11.

Alvarez-Olmos, M. I., and R. A. Oberhelman. "Probiotic Agents and Infectious Diseases: A Modern Perspective on a Traditional Therapy." *Clin Infect Dis* 32 (2001): 1567–1576.

Amaducci, L. "Phosphatidylserine in the Treatment of Alzheimer's Disease: Results of a Multicenter Study." *Psychopharmacol Bull* 24 (1988): 130–134.

Ammon, H. P., et al. "Mechanism of Anti-Inflammatory Actions of Curcumine and Boswellic Acids." *J Ethnopharmacol* 38 (1993): 113–119.

Anderson, R. A., et al. "Chromium Supplementation of Human Subjects: Effects on Glucose, Insulin, and Lipid Variables." *Metabolism* 32 (1983): 894–899.

Anderson, R. A., et al. "Elevated Intakes of Supplemental Chromium Improve Glucose and Insulin Variables in Individuals With Type 2 Diabetes." *Diabetes* 46 (1997): 1786–1791.

Arjmandi, B. H., et al. "Bone-Sparing Effect of Soy Protein in Ovarian Hormone-Deficient Rats Is Relevant to Its Isoflavone Content." *Am J Clin Nutr* 68 (1998): 1364–1368.

Arruzazabala, M. L., et al. "Comparative Study of Policosanol, Aspirin and the Combination Therapy Policosanol-Aspirin on Platelet Aggregation in Healthy Volunteers." *Pharmacol Res* 36 (1997): 293–297.

Arvill, A., and L. Bodin. "Effect of Short-Term Ingestion of Konjac Glucomannan on Serum Cholesterol in Healthy Men." *Am J Clin Nutr* 61 (1995): 585–589.

Aviram, M., et al. "Pomegranate Juice Consumption Reduces Oxidative Stress, Atherogenic Modifications to LDL, and Platelet Aggregation: Studies in Humans and in Atherosclerotic Apolipoprotein E-Deficient Mice." *Am J Clin Nutr* 71 (2000): 1062–1076.

Badmaev, V., S. Prakash and M. Majeed. "Vanadium: A Review of Its Potential Role in the Fight Against Diabetes." *J Altern Complement Med* 5 (1999): 273–291.

Bai, D. L., X. C. Tang and X. C. He. "Huperzine A, a Potential Therapeutic Agent for Treatment of Alzheimer's Disease." *Curr Med Chem* 7 (2000): 355–374.

Baird, D. D., et al. "Dietary Intervention Study to Assess Estrogenicity of Dietary Soy Among Postmenopausal Women." *J Clin Endocrinol Metab* 80 (1995): 1685–1690.

Bajendran, S., et al. "Effects of Tincture of Crataegus on the LDL Receptor Activity of Hepatic Plasma Membrane of Rats Fed an Atherogenic Diet." *Atherosclerosis* 123 (1996): 235–241.

Balestreri, R., L. Fontana and F. Astengo. "A Double-Blind Placebo Controlled Evaluation of the Safety and Efficacy of Vinpocetine in the Treatment of Patients With Chronic Vascular Senile Cerebral Dysfunction." *J Am Geriatr Soc* 35 (1987): 425–430.

Barnes, S. "Effect of Genistein on In Vitro and In Vivo Models of Cancer." *J Nutr* 125 (1995): 777–783.

———. "Evolution of the Health Benefits of Soy Isoflavones." *Proc Soc Exp Biol Med* 217 (1998): 386–392.

Barnes, S., et al. "Soybeans Inhibit Mammary Tumor Growth in Models of Breast Cancer." In *Mutagens and Carcinogens in the Diet,* edited by M. W. Pariza, 239–253. New York: Wiley Liss, 1990.

Barnes, S., T. G. Peterson and L. Coward. "Rationale for the Use of

Genistein-Containing Soy Matrices in Chemoprevention Trials for Breast and Prostate Cancer." *J Cell Biochem Suppl* 22 (1995): 181–187.

Baskaran, K., et al. "Antidiabetic Effect of a Leaf Extract From Gymnema Sylvestre in Non-Insulin-Dependent Diabetes Mellitus." *J Ethnopharm* 30 (1990): 295–305.

Batista, J., et al. "Effect of Policosanol on Hyperlipidemia and Coronary Heart Disease in Middle-Aged Patients. A 14-Month Pilot Study." *Int J Clin Pharmacol Ther* 57 (1996): 691–699.

Bendich, A. "Beta-Carotene and the Immune Response." *Proc Nutr Soc* 50 (1991): 263–274.

Bennett, J. C., and F. Plum, eds. *Cecil Textbook of Medicine.* 20th ed. Philadelphia: Saunders, 1996.

Berges, R. R., A. Kassen and T. Senge. "Treatment of Symptomatic Benign Prostatic Hyperplasia With Beta-Sitosterol: An 18-Month Follow-Up." *BJU Int* 85 (2000): 842–846.

Berges, R. R., et al. "Randomised, Placebo-Controlled, Double-Blind Clinical Trial of Beta-Sitosterol in Patients With Benign Prostatic Hyperplasia. Beta-Sitosterol Study Group." *Lancet* 345 (1995): 1529–1532.

Bielanski, T. E., and Z. H. Piotrowski. "Horse-Chestnut Seed Extract for Chronic Venous Insufficiency." *J Fam Pract* 48 (1999): 171–172.

Bisler, H., et al. "Effects of Horse-Chestnut Seed Extract on Transcapillary Filtration in Chronic Venous Insufficiency" [translated from German]. *Dtsch Med Wochenschr* 111 (1986): 1321–1329.

Blumenthal, M., ed. *The Complete German Commission E Monographs.* Boston: Integrative Medicine Communications, 1998.

Blumenthal, M., and C. Riggins. *Popular Herbs in the U.S. Market: Therapeutic Monographs.* Austin, TX: The American Botanical Council, 1997.

Boden, G., et al. "Effects of Vanadyl Sulfate on Carbohydrate and Lipid Metabolism in Patients With Non-Insulin-Dependent Diabetes Mellitus." *Metabolism* 45 (1996): 1130–1135.

Bono, G., et al. "Serotonin Precursors in Migraine Prophylaxis." *Adv Neurol* 33 (1982): 357–363.

Bonoczk, P., et al. "Role of Sodium Channel Inhibition in Neuroprotection: Effect of Vinpocetine." *Brain Res Bull* 53 (2000): 245–254.

Borchers, A. T., et al. "Mushrooms, Tumors, and Immunity." *Proc Soc Exp Biol Med* 221 (1999): 281–293.

"Boswellia Serrata." *Altern Med Rev* 3 (1998): 306–307.

Breza, J., et al. "Efficacy and Acceptability of Tadenan (Pygeum Africanum Extract) in the Treatment of Benign Prostatic Hyperplasia (BPH): A Multicentre Trial in Central Europe." *Curr Med Res Opin* 14 (1998): 127–139.

Brichard, S. M., and J. C. Henquin. "The Role of Vanadium in the Management of Diabetes." *Trends Pharmacol Sci* 16 (1995): 265–270.

Brinkeborn, R. M., D. V. Shah and F. H. Degenring. "Echinaforce and Other Echinacea Fresh Plant Preparations in the Treatment of the Common Cold. A Randomized, Placebo Controlled, Double-Blind Clinical Trial." *Phytomedicine* 6 (1999): 1–6.

Byerley, W. F., et al. "5-Hydroxytryptophan: A Review of Its Antidepressant Efficacy and Adverse Effects." *J Clin Psychopharmacol* 7 (1987): 127–137.

Byers, T., and N. Guerrero. "Epidemiologic Evidence for Vitamin C and Vitamin E in Cancer Prevention." *Am J Clin Nutr* 62 (1995): 1385–1392.

Camps, P., et al. "Huprine X Is a Novel High-Affinity Inhibitor of Acetylcholinesterase That Is of Interest for Treatment of Alzheimer's Disease." *Mol Pharmacol* 57 (2000): 409–417.

Canetti, M., et al. "A Two-Year Study on the Efficacy and Tolerability of Policosanol in Patients With Type II Hyperlipoproteinaemia." *Int J Clin Pharmacol Res* 15 (1995): 159–165.

Cangiano, C., et al. "Eating Behavior and Adherence to Dietary Prescriptions in Obese Adult Subjects Treated With 5-Hydroxytryptophan." *Am J Clin Nutr* 56 (1992): 863–867.

Cangiano, C., et al. "Effects of Oral 5-Hydroxytryptophan on Energy Intake and Macronutrient Selection in Non-Insulin Dependent Diabetic Patients." *Int J Obes Relat Metab Disord* 22 (1998): 648–654.

Carbin, B. E., B. Larsson and O. Lindahl. "Treatment of Benign Prostatic Hyperplasia With Phytosterols." *Br J Urol* 66 (1990): 639–641.

Castano, G., et al. "A Double-Blind, Placebo-Controlled Study of the Effects of Policosanol in Patients With Intermittent Claudication." *Angiology* 50 (1999): 123–130.

Ceci, F., et al. "The Effects of 5-Hydroxytryptophan Administration on Feeding Behavior in Obese Adult Female Subjects." *J Neural Transm* 76 (1989): 109–117.

Chandra, D., and S. S. Gupta. "Anti-Inflammatory and Anti-Arthritic Activity of Volatile Oil of Curcuma Longa (Haldi)." *Indian J Med Res* 60 (1972): 138–142.

Chandra, R. K. "Effect of Vitamin and Trace-Element Supplementation on Immune Responses and Infection in Elderly Subjects." *Lancet* 340 (1992): 1124–1127.

———. "Graying of the Immune System." *JAMA* 277 (1997): 1398–1399.

———. "Nutrition and the Immune System: An Introduction." *Am J Clin Nutr* 66 (1997): 460–463.

Clark, L. C., and G. F. J. Combs. "Selenium Compounds and the Prevention of Cancer: Research Needs and Public Health Implications." *J Nutr* 116 (1986): 170–173.

Clark, L. C., et al. "Effects of Selenium Supplementation for Cancer Prevention in Patients With Carcinoma of the Skin. A Randomized Controlled Trial. Nutritional Prevention of Cancer Study Group" [published erratum appears in *JAMA* 277 (May 21, 1997): 1520]. *JAMA* 276 (1996): 1957–1963.

Cline, J. M., and C. L. J. Hughes. "Phytochemicals for the Prevention of Breast and Endometrial Cancer." *Cancer Treat Res* 94 (1998): 107–134.

Colditz, G. A., and A. L. Frazier. "Models of Breast Cancer Show That Risk Is Set by Events of Early Life: Prevention Efforts Must Shift Focus." *Cancer Epiemiol Biomarkers Prev* 4 (1995): 567–571.

Cooke, J., et al. "Dietary L-L-Arginine Supplementation Normalizes Platelet Aggregation in Hypercholesterolemic Humans." *J Am Coll Card* 29 (1997): 479–485.

Crissinger, K. D., P. R. Kvietys and D. N. Granger. "Pathophysiology of Gastrointestinal Mucosal Permeability." *J Intern Med Suppl* 732 (1990): 145–154.

Crook, T. H. "Treatment of Age-Related Cognitive Decline: Effects of Phosphatidylserine." In *Anti-Aging Medical Therapeutics,* volume II, 20–29. Marina Del Ray, CA: Healthquest, 1998.

Daviglus, M. L., et al. "Fish Consumption and the 30-Year Risk of Myocardial Infarction." *New Eng J Med* 336 (1997): 1046.

De Giorgis, G., et al. "Headache in Association With Sleep Disorders in Children: A Psychodiagnostic Evaluation and Controlled Clinical Study—L 5-HTP Versus Placebo." *Drugs Exp Clin Res* 13 (1987): 425–433.

De Simone, C., et al. "The Role of Probiotics in Modulation of the Immune System in Man and in Animals." *Int J Immunother* 9 (1993): 23–28.

Deal, C. L., and R. W. Moskowitz. "Nutraceuticals As Therapeutic Agents in Osteoarthritis: The Role of Glucosamine, Chondroitin Sulfate, and Collagen Hydrolysate." *Rheum Dis Clin North Am* 25 (1999): 379–395.

Dew, M. J. "Peppermint Oil for the Irritable Bowel Syndrome: A Multicentre Trial." *British J Clin Prac* 38 (1984): 394–398.

Diehm, C., et al. "Comparison of Leg Compression Stocking and Oral Horse-Chestnut Seed Extract Therapy in Patients With Chronic Venous Insufficiency." *Lancet* 347 (1996): 292–294.

Doi, K., et al. "Treatment of Diabetes With Glucomannan (Konjac Mannan)." *Lancet* (1979): 987–988.

Elliott, R. B., et al. "A Population Based Strategy to Prevent Insulin-Dependent Diabetes Using Nicotinamide." *J Pediatr Endocrinol Metab* 9 (1996): 501–509.

Fraker, P. J., et al. "Interrelationships Between Zinc and Immune Function." *Fed Proc* 45 (1986): 1474–1479.

Fund, W. C. R. *Food, Nutrition, and the Prevention of Cancer: A Global Perspective.* Washington, DC: American Institute Cancer Research, 1997.

Gandini, S., et al. "Meta-Analysis of Studies on Breast Cancer Risk and Diet: The Role of Fruit and Vegetable Consumption and the Intake of Associated Micronutrients." *Eur J Cancer* 36 (2000): 636–646.

Garland, M., et al. "Antioxidant Micronutrients and Breast Cancer." *J Am Coll Nutr* 12 (1993): 400–411.

Gerber, G. S., et al. "Saw Palmetto (Serenoa Repens) in Men With Lower Urinary Tract Symptoms: Effects on Urodynamic Parameters and Voiding Symptoms." *Urology* 51 (1998): 1003–1007.

Gilbert, G. J. "Ginkgo Biloba." *Neurology* 48 (1997): 1137.

Gionchetti, P., et al. "Probiotics in Infective Diarrhea and Inflammatory Bowel Diseases." *J Gastroenterol Hepatol* 15 (2000): 489–493.

Godhwani, S., J. L. Godhwani and D. S. Vyas. "Ocimum Sanctum: An Experimental Study Evaluating Its Anti-Inflammatory, Analgesic and Antipyretic Activity in Animals." *J Ethnopharmacol* 21 (1987): 153–163.

Gordon, M., et al. "A Placebo-Controlled Trial of the Immune Modulator, Lentinan, in HIV-Positive Patients: A Phase I/II Trial." *J Med* 29 (1998): 305–330.

Graham, I., et al. "Plasma Homocysteine As a Risk Factor for Vascular Disease." *JAMA* 277 (1997): 1775–1781.

Graham, S., et al. "Nutritional Epidemiology of Postmenopausal Breast Cancer in Western New York." *Am J Epidemiol* 134 (1991): 552–566.

Gunning, K., and P. Steele. "Echinacea for the Prevention of Upper Respiratory Tract Infections." *J Fam Pract* 48 (1999): 93.

Halberstam, M., et al. "Oral Vanadyl Sulfate Improves Insulin Sensitivity in NIDDM but Not in Obese Nondiabetic Subjects." *Diabetes* 45 (1996): 659–666.

Harvard Medical School, Health Publications Group. "A Special Report: High Blood Pressure." *Harvard Health Letter* (1990).

Hernandez, F., et al. "Effect of Policosanol on Serum Lipids and Lipoproteins in Healthy Volunteers." *Curr Therapeutic Res* 51 (1992): 568–575.

Hirano, T., M. Homma and K. Oka. "Effects of Stinging Nettle Root Extracts and Their Steroidal Components on the Na+,K(+)-ATPase of the Benign Prostatic Hyperplasia." *Planta Med* 60 (1994): 30–33.

Hirasawa, M., et al. "Three Kinds of Antibacterial Substances From Lentinus Edodes (Berk.) Sing. (Shiitake, an Edible Mushroom)." *Int J Antimicrob Agents* 11 (1999): 151–157.

Hirata, J. D., et al. "Does Dong Quai Have Estrogenic Effects in Postmenopausal Women? A Double-Blind, Placebo-Controlled Trial." *Fertil Steril* 68 (1997): 981–986.

Hirayama, K., and J. Rafter. "The Role of Probiotic Bacteria in Cancer Prevention." *Microbes Infect* 2 (2000): 681–686.

Hishida, I., H. Nanba and H. Kuroda. "Antitumor Activity Exhibited by Orally Administered Extract From Fruit Body of *Grifola Frondosa* (Maitake)." *Clin Pharm Bull* (Tokyo).

Hou, Y. D., et al. "Effect of *Radix Astragali* Seu Hedysari on the Interferon System." *Chin Med J* (Engl) 94 (1981): 35–40.

Hryb, D. J., et al. "The Effect of Extracts of the Roots of the Stinging Nettle (Urtica Dioica) on the Interaction of SHBG With Its Receptor on Human Prostatic Membranes." *Planta Med* 61 (1995): 31–32.

Hunter, D. J., and W. C. Willett. "Nutrition and Breast Cancer." *Cancer Causes Control* 7 (1996): 56–68.

Imai, K., and K. Nakachi. "Cross Sectional Study of Effects of Drinking Green Tea on Cardiovascular and Liver Diseases." *BMJ* 310 (1995): 693–696.

Ingram, D., et al. "Case-Control Study of Phytoestrogens and Breast Cancer." *Lancet* 350 (1997): 990–994.

Jones, K. "Shiitake: A Major Medicinal Mushroom." *Alt Compl Ther* 4 (1998): 53–59.

Kahn, R. S., et al. "Effect of a Serotonin Precursor and Uptake Inhibitor in Anxiety Disorders: A Double-Blind Comparison of 5-Hydroxy-tryptophan, Clomipramine and Placebo." *Int Clin Psychopharmacol* 2 (1987): 33–45.

Kanowski, S., et al. "Proof of Efficacy of the *Ginkgo Biloba* Special Extract E Gb 761 in Outpatients Suffering From Mild to Moderate Primary Degenerative Dementia of the Alzheimer Type or Multi-Infarct Dementia." *Pharmacopsychiatry* 29 (1996): 47–56.

Kariya, Y., et al. "Occurrence of Chondroitin Sulfate E in Glycosamino Isolated From the Body Wall of Sea Cucumber Stichopus Japonicus." *J Biol Chem* 265 (1990): 50–55.

Kawano, Y., et al. "Effects of Magnesium Supplementation in Hypertensive Patients: Assessment by Office, Home, and Ambulatory Blood Pressures." *Hypertension* 32 (1999): 260–265.

Kelly, G. S. "The Role of Glucosamine Sulfate and Chondroitin Sulfates in the Treatment of Degenerative Joint Disease." *Altern Med Rev* 3 (1998): 27–39.

Kelm, M. A., et al. "Antioxidant and Cyclooxygenase Inhibitory Phenolic Compounds From Ocimum Sanctum Linn." *Phytomedicine* 7 (2000): 7–13.

Kennedy, A. R. "The Evidence for Soybean Products As Cancer Preventive Agents." *J Nutr* 125 (1995): 733–743.

Khaw, K. "Dietary Potassium and Stroke Associated Mortality." *New Eng J Med* 216 (1987): 235–240.

Kidd, P. M. "The Use of Mushroom Glucans and Proteoglycans in Cancer Treatment." *Altern Med Rev* 5 (2000): 4–27.

Kleijnen, J., and P. Knipschild. "Ginkgo Biloba for Cerebral Insufficiency." *Br J Clin Pharmacol* 34 (1992): 352–358.

Klepser, T., and N. Nisly. "Astragalus As an Adjunctive Therapy in Immunocompromised Patients." *Alt Med Alert* (Nov. 1999): 125–128.

Klippel, K. F., D. M. Hiltl and B. Schipp. "A Multicentric, Placebo-Controlled, Double-Blind Clinical Trial of Beta-Sitosterol

(Phytosterol) for the Treatment of Benign Prostatic Hyperplasia. German BPH-Phyto Study Group." *B J Urol* 80 (1997): 427–432.

Kono, S., et al. "Green Tea Consumption and Serum Lipid Profiles: A Cross-Sectional Study in Northern Kyushu, Japan." *Prev Med* 21 (1992): 526–531.

Konrad, T., et al. "Alpha Lipoic Acid Treatment Decreases Serum Lactate and Pyruvate Concentrations and Improves Glucose Effectiveness in Lean and Obese Patients With Type 2 Diabetes." *Diabetes Care* 22 (1999): 280–287.

Kopp-Hoolihan, L. "Prophylactic and Therapeutic Uses of Probiotics: A Review." *J Am Diet Assoc* 101 (2001): 229–238.

Krishna, G. C. "Increased Blood Pressure During Potassium Depletion in Normotensive Men." *New Eng J Med* 329 (1989): 1177–1182.

Krzeski, T., et al. "Combined Extracts of Urtica Dioica and Pygeum Africanum in the Treatment of Benign Prostatic Hyperplasia: Double-Blind Comparison of Two Doses." *Clin Ther* 15 (1993): 1011–1020.

Kulkarni, R. R., et al. "Treatment of Osteoarthritis With a Herbomineral Formulation: A Double-Blind, Placebo-Controlled, Cross-Over Study." *J Ethnopharmacol* 33 (1991): 91–95.

Kushi, L. H., et al. "Dietary Antioxidant Vitamins and Death From Coronary Heart Disease in Postmenopausal Women." *N Engl J Med* 334 (1996): 1156–1162.

Landrum, et al. "A One-Year Study of the Macular Pigment: The Effect of 140 Days of a Lutein Supplement." *Exp Eye Res* 65 (1997): 57–62.

Langsjoen, P., et al. "Treatment of Essential Hypertension With Coenzyme Q_{10}." *Molec Asp Med* 15 (1994): 265–272.

Lansky, E. "Pomegranate Seed Oil Triggers Self-Destruct Mechanism in Breast Cancer Cells." Technion-Israel Institute of Technology. Paper presented in Madrid, June 2001.

Law, M. R. "By How Much Does Dietary Salt Reduction Lower Blood Pressure?" *Brit Med J* 302 (1991): 819–924.

Le Bars, P. L., et al. "A Placebo-Controlled, Double-Blind, Randomized Trial of an Extract of *Ginkgo Biloba* for Dementia. North American E Gb Study Group." *JAMA* 278 (1997): 1327–1332.

Lee, H. P., et al. "Dietary Effects on Breast-Cancer Risk in Singapore." *Lancet* 337 (1991): 1197–1200.

Leicester, R. "Peppermint Oil to Reduce Colonic Spasm During Endoscopy." *Lancet II* (1982): 989.

Lichius, J. J., and C. Muth. "The Inhibiting Effects of Urtica Dioica Root Extracts on Experimentally Induced Prostatic Hyperplasia in the Mouse." *Planta Med* 63 (1997): 307–310.

Lieberman, S. "A Review of the Effectiveness of *Cimicifuga Racemosa* (Black Cohosh) for the Symptoms of Menopause." *J Womens Health* 5 (1998): 525–529.

Lima, M., et al. "The Effect of Magnesium Supplementation in Increasing Doses on the Control of Type 2 Diabetes." *Diabetes Care* 21 (1998): 682–686.

Loschen, G., and L. Ebeling. "Inhibition of Arachidonic Acid Cascade by Extract of Rye Pollen." *Arzneimittelforschung* 41 (1991): 162–167.

Lotz-Winter, H. "On the Pharmacology of Bromelain: An Update With Special Regard to Animal Studies on Dose-Dependent Effects." *Planta Med* 56 (1990): 249–253.

Lowe, F. C., et al. "Review of Recent Placebo-Controlled Trials Utilizing Phytotherapeutic Agents for Treatment of BPH." *Prostate* 37 (1998): 187–193.

Lyle, et al. "Antioxidant Intake and Risk of Incident Age-Related Nuclear Cataracts in the Beaver Dam Eye Study." *Am J Epidemiol* 149 (1999): 801–809.

MacDonald, R., et al. "A Systematic Review of Cernilton for the Treatment of Benign Prostatic Hyperplasia." *BJU Int* 85 (2000): 836–841.

Madar, Z., et al. "Glucose-Lowering Effect of Fenugreek in Non-Insulin Dependent Diabetics." *Eur J Clin Nutr* 42 (1988): 51–54.

Maebashi, M., et al. "Therapeutic Evaluation of the Effect of Biotin on Hyperglycemia in Patients With Non-Insulin Dependent Diabetes Mellitus." *J Clin Biochem Nutr* 14 (1993): 211–218.

Marchioli, R. "Antioxidant Vitamins and Prevention of Cardiovascular Disease: Laboratory, Epidemiological and Clinical Trial Data." *Pharmacol Res* 40 (1999): 227–238.

Mares-Perlman, et al. "Lutein and Zeaxanthin in the Diet and Serum and Their Relation to Age-Related Maculopathy in the Third National Health and Nutrition Examination Survey." *Am J Epid* 153 (2001): 424–432.

Margretts, J. B. "Mortality Patterns Among Hypertensives by Reported

Level of Caffeine Consumption." *Preventive Medicine* 17 (1988): 310–320.

Mas, R., et al. "Effects of Policosanol in Patients With Type II Hypercholesterolemia and Additional Coronary Risk Factors." *Clin Pharmacol Ther* 65 (1999): 439–447.

Mas, R., et al. "Pharmacoepidemiologic Study of Policosanol." *Curr Ther Res* 60 (1999): 458–467.

Mathe, G., et al. "A Pygeum Africanum Extract With So-Called Phyto-Estrogenic Action Markedly Reduces the Volume of True and Large Prostatic Hypertrophy." *Biomed Pharmacother* 49 (1995): 341–343.

Mayell, M. "Maitake Extracts and Their Therapeutic Potential." *Altern Med Rev* 6 (2001): 48–60.

McAlindon, T. E., et al. "Glucosamine and Chondroitin for Treatment of Osteoarthritis: A Systematic Quality Assessment and Meta-Analysis." *JAMA* 283 (2000): 1469–1475.

McCully, K. S. "Homocysteine and Vascular Disease." *Nat Med* 2 (1996): 386–389.

Melchart, D., et al. "Echinacea Root Extracts for the Prevention of Respiratory Tract Infections: A Double-Blind, Placebo-Controlled Randomized Trial." *Arch Fam Med* 7 (1998): 541–545.

Menchini-Fabris, G. F., et al. "New Perspectives on the Use of Pygeum Africanum in Prostato-Bladder Pathology." *Arch Ital Urol Nefrol Androl* 60 (1988): 313–322.

Messina, M. J., V. Persky and K. D. Setchell. "Soy Intake and Cancer Risk: A Review of the *In Vitro* and *In Vivo* Data." *Nutr Cancer* 21 (1994): 113–131.

Messina, M., S. Barnes and K. D. Setchell. "Phyto-Estrogens and Breast Cancer." *Lancet* 350 (1997): 971–972.

Mizuno, M. "Anti-Tumor Polysaccharides From Mushrooms During Storage." *Biofactors* 12 (2000): 275–281.

Mowrey, D. B. "Motion Sickness, Ginger, and Psychophysics." *Lancet* I (1982): 655–657.

Muth, E. R., J. M. Laurent and P. Jasper. "The Effect of Bilberry Nutritional Supplementation on Night Visual Acuity and Contrast Sensitivity." *Alt Med Rev* 5 (2000): 164–173.

Nachtigall, L. B., et al. "The Effects of Isoflavones Derived From Red Clover on Vasomotor Symptoms and Endometrial Thickness. 9th International Menopause Society World Congress on the Menopause. October 17–21, 1999.

Nair, M. G. "MSU Study: Tart Cherries a Pain Killer." *J Natl Products* (2000).

Nanba, H. "Antitumor Activity of Orally Administered 'D-Fraction' From Maitake Mushroom (Grifola Frondosa)." *J Naturopathic Med* 4 (1993): 10–15.

———. "Immunostimulant Activity In Vivo and Anti-HIV Activity In Vitro of 3 Branched b–1–6 Glucans Extracted From Maitake Mushrooms *(Grifola Frondosa)*." VIII International Conference on AIDS, Amsterdam, 1992.

Nanba, H., A. Hamaguchi and H. Kuroda. "The Chemical Structure of an Antitumor Polysaccharide in Fruit Bodies of *Grifola Frondosa* (Maitake)." *Chem Pharm Bull* 35 (Tokyo) (1987): 1162–1168.

Nanba, H., and H. Kuroda. "Antitumor Mechanisms of Orally Administered Shiitake Fruit Bodies." *Chem Pharm Bull* 35 (Tokyo) (1987): 2459–2464.

Niewoehner, C. B., et al. "Role of Zinc Supplementation in Type II Diabetes Mellitus." *Am J Med* 81 (1986): 63–68.

North American Menopause Society. "The Role of Isoflavones in Menopausal Health: Consensus of the North American Menopause Society." *Menopause* 7 (2000): 215–229.

Ornish, D., et al. "Can Lifestyle Changes Reverse Coronary Heart Disease?" *Lancet* 336 (1990): 129–133.

Otomo, E., et al. "Comparison of Vinpocetine With Ifenprodil Tartrate and Dihydroergotoxine Mesylate Treatment and Results of Long-Term Treatment With Vinpocetine." *Curr Therapeutic Res* 37 (1985): 811–821.

Paolisso, G., et al. "Improved Insulin Response and Action by Chronic Magnesium Administration in Aged NIDDM Subjects." *Diabetes Care* 12 (1989): 265–269.

Patki, P. S. "Efficacy of Potassium and Magnesium in Essential Hypertension: A Double-Blind, Placebo-Controlled, Crossover Study." *B Med Journ* 301 (1990): 521–523.

Persaud, S. J., et al. "Gymnema Sylvestre Stimulates Insulin Release In Vitro by Increased Membrane Permeability." *J Endocrinol* 163 (1999): 207–212.

Peterson, G., and S. Barnes. "Genistein Inhibits Both Estrogen and Growth Factor-Stimulated Proliferation of Human Breast Cancer Cells." *Cell Growth Differ* 7 (1996): 1345–1351.

Pittler, M. H., and E. Ernst. "Horse-Chestnut Seed Extract for Chronic Venous Insufficiency. A Criteria-Based Systematic Review." *Arch Dermatol* 134 (1998): 1356–1360.

Poldinger, W., B. Calanchini and W. Schwarz. "A Functional–Dimensional Approach to Depression: Serotonin Deficiency As a Target Syndrome in a Comparison of 5-Hydroxytryptophan and Fluvoxamine." *Psychopathology* 24 (1991): 53–81.

Polo, V., A. Saibene and A. E. Pontiroli. "Nicotinamide Improves Insulin Secretion and Metabolic Control in Lean Type 2 Diabetic Patients With Secondary Failure to Sulphonylureas." *Acta Diabetol* 35 (1998): 61–64.

Pons, P., et al. "Effects of Policosanol in Elderly Hypercholesterolemic Patients." *Curr Th* 53 (1993): 265–269.

Quella, S. K., et al. "Evaluation of Soy Phytoestrogens for the Treatment of Hot Flashes in Breast Cancer Survivors: A North Central Cancer Treatment Group Trial." *J Clin Oncon* 18 (2000): 1068–1074.

Qureshi, A. A., et al. "Lowering of Serum Cholesterol in Hyper-cholesterolemic Humans by Tocotrienols (Palmvitee)." *Am J Clin Nutr* 53 (1991): 1021–1026.

Rees, W. "Treating Irritable Bowel Syndrome With Peppermint Oil." *Br Med J II* (1979): 835–836.

Reginster, J. Y., et al. "A Randomized Placebo Controlled Clinical Trial on the Long-Term Effects of Glucosamine Sulphate on Osteoarthritis Progression." *Lancet* 357 (2001): 251–256.

Reisin, E. "Effect of Weight Loss Without Salt Restriction on the Reduction of Blood Pressure in Overweight Hypertensive Patients." *New Eng J Med* 298 (1978): 1–6.

Reljanovic, M., et al. "Treatment of Diabetic Polyneuropathy With the Antioxidant Thioctic Acid (Alpha-Lipoic Acid): A Two-Year Multicenter Randomized Double-Blind Placebo-Controlled Trial (ALADIN II). Alpha Lipoic Acid in Diabetic Neuropathy." *Free Radic Res* 31 (1999): 171–179.

Rimm, E. B., et al. "Antioxidants for Vascular Disease." *Med Clin North Am* 84 (2000): 239–249.

Rimm, E. B., et al. "Folate and Vitamin B$_6$ From Diet and Supplements in Relation to Risk of Coronary Heart Disease Among Women." *JAMA* 279 (1998): 359–364.

Rimm, E. B., et al. "Vitamin E Consumption and the Risk of Coronary Heart Disease in Men." *N Engl J Med* 328 (1993): 1450–1456.

Rosenberg, I. H., and J. W. Miller. "Nutritional Factors in Physical and Cognitive Functions of Elderly People." *American Journal of Clinical Nutrition* 55 (1992): 1237–1243.

Sacks, F. M. "Dietary Fats and Blood Pressure: A Critical Review of the Evidence." *Nutrition Reviews* 47 (1989): 291–300.

Sano, M., et al. "Effect of Tea (Camellia Sinensis L.) on Lipid Peroxidation in Rat Liver and Kidney: A Comparison of Green and Black Tea Feeding." *Biol Pharm Bull* 18 (1995): 1006–1008.

Santos, M. S., et al. "Natural Killer Cell Activity in Elderly Men Is Enhanced by Beta-Carotene Supplementation." *Am J Clin Nutr* 64 (1996): 772–777.

Schelber, M. D., and R. W. Rebar. "Isoflavones and Postmenopausal Bone Health: A Viable Alternative to Estrogen Therapy." *Menopause* 6 (1999): 233–241.

Seddon, et al. "Dietary Carotenoids, Vitamin A, C and E, and Advanced Age-Related Macular Degeneration. Eye Disease Case-Control Study Group." *JAMA* 272 (1994): 1413–1420.

Segars, L.W. "Saw Palmetto Extracts for Benign Prostatic Hyperplasia." *J Fam Pract* 48 (1999): 88–89.

Selhub, J., et al. "Vitamin Status and Intake As Primary Determinants of Homocysteinemia in an Elderly Population." *JAMA* 270 (1993): 2693–2698.

Semba, R. D. "Vitamin A, Immunity, and Infection." *Clin Infect* Dis 19 (1994): 489–499.

Serafini, M., A. Ghiselli and A. Ferro-Luzzi. "In Vivo Antioxidant Effect of Green and Black Tea in Man." *Eur J Clin Nutr* 50 (1996): 28–32.

Shanmugasundaram, E. R., et al. "Use of Gymnema Sylvestre Leaf Extract in the Control of Blood Glucose in Insulin-Dependent Diabetes Mellitus." *J Ethnopharmacol* 30 (1990): 281–294.

Sharma, R. D., T. C. Raghuram and N. S. Rao. "Effect of Fenugreek Seeds on Blood Glucose and Serum Lipids in Type 1 Diabetes." *Eur J Clin Nutr* 44 (1990): 301–306.

Simon and Hudes. "Serum Ascorbic Acid and Other Correlates of Self-Reported Cataract Among Older Americans." *J Clin Epidmiol* 52 (1999): 207–211.

Sinatra, S. T. "Coenzyme Q$_{10}$: A Vital Therapeutic Nutrient for the Heart With Special Application in Congestive Heart Failure." *Conn Med* 61 (1997): 707–711.

Singh, S., D. K. Majumdar and H. M. Rehan. "Evaluation of Anti-Inflammatory Potential of Fixed Oil of Ocimum Sanctum (Holybasil) and Its Possible Mechanism of Action." *J Ethnopharmacol* 54 (1996): 19–26.

Stensvold, I., et al. "Tea Consumption. Relationship to Cholesterol, Blood Pressure, and Coronary and Total Mortality." *Prev Med* 21 (1992): 546–553.

Stoll, B. A. "Eating to Beat Breast Cancer: Potential Role for Soy Supplements." *Ann Oncol* 8 (1997): 223–225.

Stusser, R., et al. "Long-Term Therapy With Policosanol Improves Treadmill Exercise-ECG Testing Performance of Coronary Heart Disease Patients." *Int J Clin Pharmacol Ther* 36 (1998): 469–473.

Sun, Q. Q., et al. "Huperzine-A Capsules Enhance Memory and Learning Performance in 34 Pairs of Matched Adolescent Students" [abstract]. *Chung Kuo Yao Li Hsueh Pao* 20 (1999): 601–603.

Sun, Y., et al. "Immune Restoration and/or Augmentation of Local Graft Versus Host Reaction by Traditional Chinese Medicinal Herbs." *Cancer* 52 (1983): 70–73.

Taguchi, I. "Clinical Efficacy of Lentinan on Patients With Stomach Cancer: End Points Results of a Four-Year Follow-Up Survey." *Cancer Detect Prevent Suppl* 1 (1987): 333–349.

Taussig, S. J., and S. Batkin. "Bromelain, the Enzyme Complex of Pineapple (Ananas Comosus) and Its Clinical Application. An Update." *J Ethnopharmacol* 22 (1988): 191–203.

Taylor, M. "Alternatives to Hormone Replacement Therapy." *Comprehensive Therapy* 23 (1997): 514–532.

Teikari, et al. "Long-Term Supplementation With Alpha-Tocopherol and Beta-Carotene and Age-Related Cataract." *Acta Ophthalmol Scand* 75 (1997): 634–640.

Thacker, H. L., and D. L. Booher. "Management of Perimenopause: Focus on Alternative Therapies." *Cleveland Clin J Med* 66 (1999): 213–218.

Thomas, S. R., et al. "Inhibition of LDL Oxidation by Ubiquinol-10. A Protective Mechanism for Coenzyme Q10 in Atherogenesis?" *Molec Asp Med* 18, supplement (1997): 85–103.

Tomeo, A. C., et al. "Antioxidant Effects of Tocotrienols in Patients With Hyperlipidemia and Carotid Stenosis." *Lipids* 30 (1995): 1179–1183.

Van Dongen, M. C., et al. "The Efficacy of Ginkgo for Elderly People With Dementia and Age-Associated Memory Impairment: New Results of a Randomized Clinical Trial." *J Am Geriatr Soc* 48 (2000): 1183–1194.

Ved, H. S., et al. "Huperzine A, a Potential Therapeutic Agent for Dementia, Reduces Neuronal Cell Death Caused by Glutamate." *Neuroreport* 8 (1997): 963–968.

Venter, C. S., et al. "The Effects of Dietary Fiber Component Konjac-Glucomannan on Serum Cholesterol Levels of Hypercholesterolemic Subjects." *Hum Nutr Food Sci Nutr* 41 (1987): 55–61.

Vieira, R. P., C. Pedrosa and P. A. Mourao. "Extensive Heterogeneity of Proteoglycans Bearing Fucose-Branched Chondroitin Sulfate Extracted From the Connective Tissue of Sea Cucumber." *Biochemistry* 32 (1993): 2254–2262.

Vuksan, V., et al. "Konjac-Mannan (Glucomannan) Improves Glycemia and Other Associated Risk Factors for Coronary Heart Disease in Type 2 Diabetes. A Randomized Controlled Metabolic Trial." *Diabetes Care* 22 (1999): 913–919.

Wang, H., et al. "Novel Antioxidant Compounds From Tart Cherries (Prunus Cerasus)." *J Nat Prod* 62 (1999): 86–88.

Warnecke, G. "Influencing Menopausal Symptoms With a Phytotherapeutic Agent: Successful Therapy With *Cimicifuga* Mono-Extract." *Med Welt* 36 (1985): 871–874.

Weikl, A., et al. "Crataegus Special Extract WS 1442. Assessment of Objective Effectiveness in Patients With Heart Failure." *Fortschritte Der Medizin* 114 (1996): 291–296.

Whelton, P. K. "Sodium Reduction and Weight Loss in the Treatment of Hypertension in Older Persons." *JAMA* 279 (1998): 839–846.

Wilt, T. J., et al. "Saw Palmetto Extracts for Treatment of Benign Prostatic Hyperplasia: A Systematic Review." *JAMA* 280 (1998): 1604–1609.

Wilt, T. J., R. MacDonald and A. Ishani. "Beta-Sitosterol for the Treatment of Benign Prostatic Hyperplasia: A Systematic Review." *BJU Int* 83 (1999): 976–983.

Xu, S. S., et al. "Efficacy of Tablet Huperzine-A on Memory, Cognition, and Behavior in Alzheimer's Disease." *Chung Kuo Yao Li Hsueh Pao* 16 (1995): 391–395.

Yamada, Y., H. Nanba and H. Kuroda. "Antitumor Effect of Orally Administered Extracts From Fruit Body of *Grifola Frondosa* (Maitake)." *Chem Pharm Bull* 38 (1990): 790–796.

Zakay-Rones, Z., et al. "Inhibition of Several Strains of Influenza Virus In Vitro and Reduction of Symptoms by an Elderberry Extract (Sambucus Nigra L.) During an Outbreak of Influenza B Panama." *J Altern Complement Med* 1 (1995): 361–369.

Zhang, S., et al. "Dietary Carotenoids and Vitamins A, C, and E and Risk of Breast Cancer." *J Natl Cancer Inst* 91 (1999): 547–556.

Zhang, X., et al. "Effect of the Extracts of Pumpkinseeds on the Urodynamics of Rabbits: An Experimental Study." *J Tongji Med Univ* 14 (1994): 235–238.

Zheng, Z., et al. "Studies on Chemical Constituents and Immunological Function Activity of Hairy Root of Astragalus Membranaceus." *Chin J Biotechnol* 14 (1998): 93–97.

pasta 182
pathway to healing 2, 3, 6, 7, 9, 24, 25, 26, 34, 45, 114, 142, 154, 162, 188
Paxil 131
peace 5, 10, 24, 27, 32, 34, 35, 39, 122, 204, 205
peanut oil 118
pectin 99
peppermint vii, 105, 109, 137, 195
peppermint oil vii, 109, 137
perimenopausal 159
peripheral neuropathy 85
periwinkle 125, 126, 127
persistence 24
phosphatidylserine (PS) 126
phytoestrogen 161, 175
pineapple 117, 165
pinto beans 177
plant kingdom 7, 8, 10, 26, 50, 62, 70, 109, 116, 128, 139, 152, 171, 174, 178, 186, 187
platelets 44, 45, 48, 51, 60
platycodon 187, 190
PMS viii, 131, 166, 167, 168, 169
pneumonia 72, 100
policosanol vi, 50, 51, 53, 62
polyphenols vi, 56, 73, 185
pomegranate 70, 74
pork 13, 20, 21
potassium vi, 47, 54, 56, 57, 176, 182, 194
potatoes 182, 183, 200, 201, 202
poultry 101, 185
Pravachol 50
prayer v, 6, 7, 24, 26, 27, 29, 30, 31, 32, 33, 34, 35, 42, 45, 46, 82, 168,

205, 206
Precose 88
Premarin 163
premature supraventricular tachycardia (PSVT) 43, 44
premature ventricular contractions (PVCs) 45
premenstrual syndrome 166, 167, 168
probiotic 100, 101
progestin 158, 160, 178
Proscar 152
prostaglandins 175
prostate viii, 69, 150, 151, 152, 153, 154, 155, 156, 161, 163, 184, 196
prostate enlargement viii, 150, 151, 152, 153, 154, 155, 161
protein 21, 61, 80, 98, 103, 143, 146, 175, 182, 183, 185, 195
proteolytic enzymes 98
proton pump inhibitors 107
Provera 163
Prozac 131, 189
prunes 92, 176, 202
PSA level 155
psyllium 92, 109, 176, 177
pulse 41, 52, 108
pumpkinseed extract 154
pygeum 152, 156

Q
quercetin 80, 146, 149, 197

R
red clover 153, 154, 156, 161, 164, 175
red meat 185
reishi mushroom 71, 74
relaxation 57, 135
Reminyl 125
renal disease 86, 132

reptiles 20
respiratory infection 65, 75
resveratrol 80
retina 143, 144, 147, 148, 149
retinopathy 142, 144, 146, 147
rheumatoid arthritis 64, 66, 111, 127
rice 51, 92, 202
rice bran 51
romaine lettuce 145
rye pollen extract 153, 156

S
safflower oil 118
salmon 20, 89, 175, 185, 202
salsa 184
salt water 79
salvation 4, 5, 14, 15, 18, 33, 64, 206
saponins 175
sardines 175, 185
saturated fat 19, 48, 49, 51, 83, 118, 176, 178, 182, 183
saw palmetto 152, 155, 156
scleroderma 66
sclerotherapy 171
sea cucumber 116, 117, 120
selective serotonin reuptake inhibitors 130
selenium 61, 69, 70, 74, 78, 194
serotonin vii, 127, 129, 130, 131, 132, 133, 166, 168, 186, 189
shellfish 21, 119
shiitake mushroom 71, 75, 198
shrimp 21
side effects 26, 44, 50, 55, 56, 58, 62, 81, 91,

MORE RESOURCES FROM DR. CHERRY

Pathway to Healing medical magazine

Dr. Cherry's monthly publication sorts through the confusion about health and healing. It shares sensible, biblical and medical steps you can use to get well. Every issue points you to your pathway to healing. Writing from a Christian physician's Bible-based point of view, Dr. Cherry talks about nutrition and health, how to pray for specific diseases, updates on the latest medical research, Linda's own recipes for healthy eating, and questions and answers about issues you need to know.

God's Pathway to Healing: Digestion

Dr. Cherry discusses keys to a naturally healthy digestive system, including better digestion and absorption of food, proper elimination of waste, and the function of "good" bacteria. He points readers toward better eating habits and natural nutritional supplements to improve digestion.

God's Pathway to Healing: Joints and Arthritis

Painful joints and arthritis do not have to be part of aging, says Dr. Cherry. Recent medical breakthroughs show that natural substances can relieve pain and inflammation and slow or prevent cartilage loss.

God's Pathway to Healing: Vision

Macular degeneration, cataracts, vision deterioration due to complications of diabetes, and other eye conditions can be slowed or prevented. Dr. Cherry discusses herbs and nutritional changes you can make to keep vision strong.

Dr. Cherry's Little Instruction Book

With practical health and healing tips on every page, now you can use this helpful, concise book as a handy reference for the benefit of everyone in your family! Learn about God-given foods to improve your health, natural remedies, tips on diet and exercise, and scriptures and prayers for healing.

Study Guides, Volume 2

Dr. Cherry discusses thirty common medical conditions that friends and partners have requested specific information about—high blood pressure, chronic fatigue, fibromyalgia, IBS, MS, PMS and varicose veins—just to name a few. This informative and practical guidebook can help you prevent and reverse physical attacks against your body.

Prayers That Heal

Combining the wisdom of over twenty-five years of medical practice and the revelation of God's Word, Dr. Cherry provides the knowledge you need to pray effectively against diabetes, cancer, heart disease, eye problems, hypoglycemia and other common afflictions that try to rob you of your health.

Healing Prayer

In this fascinating, in-depth look at a vital link between spiritual and physical healing, Dr. Cherry presents case histories of people healed through prayer, plus the latest information on herbs, vitamins and supplements that promote vibrant health. This is sound information you need to keep you healthy—mind, soul and body.

God's Pathway to Healing: Prostate

Prostate disease is a rapidly growing concern, affecting nearly 250,000 men this year. Modern medicine says that all men will face prostate problems if they live long enough, but you don't have to. In this book, Dr. Cherry shows how combining God-given nutrients with Spirit-directed prayer can be God's pathway to healing—or preventing—prostate disease for you.

God's Pathway to Healing: Herbs That Heal

Dr. Cherry breaks through the bewildering maze of advertising claims and the incredible explosion of products on the shelves with this enlightening book. It's a virtual road map of what to use and what to avoid—even how to be cautious in combining herbs. God has provided plants to help combat sickness and disease—now you'll know how to use them!

God's Pathway to Helping: Menopause

This book is full of helpful advice for women who are going through what can be a very stressful time of life. Find out what foods, supplements and steps can be taken to find a pathway to healing for menopause and perimenopause. This is a practical and helpful resource for all women.

To order these books or for more information, contact:
Reginald B. Cherry Ministries
P. O. Box 27711
Houston, TX 77227
Phone: 888-372-4377
www.drcherry.org